How to Control Your BLOOD PRESSURE *for Healthy Living*

How to Control Your BLOOD PRESSURE *for Healthy Living*

By

Dr. G.D. Thapar

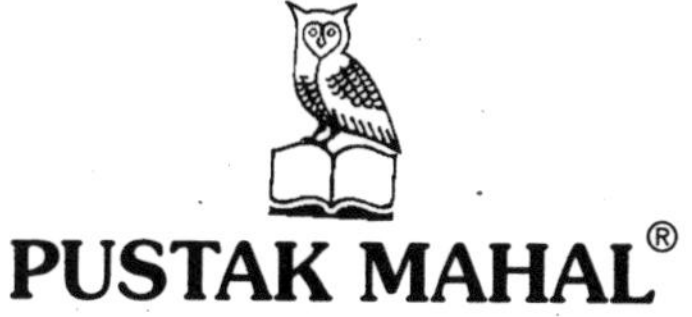

PUSTAK MAHAL®

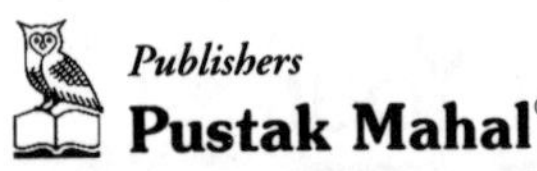
Publishers
Pustak Mahal®

J-3/16 , Daryaganj, New Delhi-110002
☎ 23276539, 23272783, 23272784 • *Fax:* 011-23260518
E-mail: info@pustakmahal.com • *Website:* www.pustakmahal.com

Sales Centre

- 10-B, Netaji Subhash Marg, Daryaganj, New Delhi-110002
  ☎ 23268292, 23268293, 23279900 • *Fax:* 011-23280567
  E-mail: rapidexdelhi@indiatimes.com
- 6686, Khari Baoli, Delhi-110006
  ☎ 23944314, 23911979

Branches

Bengaluru: ☎ 080-22234025 • *Telefax:* 080-22240209
E-mail: pustak@airtelmail.in • pustak@sancharnet.in
Mumbai: ☎ 022-22010941, 022-22053387
E-mail: rapidex@bom5.vsnl.net.in
Patna: ☎ 0612-3294193 • *Telefax:* 0612-2302719
E-mail: rapidexptn@rediffmail.com
Hyderabad: *Telefax:* 040-24737290
E-mail: pustakmahalhyd@yahoo.co.in

ISBN 978-81-223-0634-7
Edition: 2012

NOTICE

Author's Note

The information contained in this book is intended to supplement your doctor's advice and guidance. It is not meant to replace it.
Do not attempt to make your own diagnosis. Self treatment can be dangerous, especially in the case of serious illness.

Printed at : **Super Fine Book Binding Works, (U.P.)**

Dedicated to the memory
of my teacher
Prof. K.L. Wig

Preface to the Second Edition

With the addition of new material and changes in the existing chapters, the book has been brought up-to-date in line with current medical thinking on hypertension. I do hope the book will continue to help the readers improve quality of their lives.

I take this opportunity to express my sense of gratitude to my new publishers, Pustak Mahal, for taking keen interest in the production of the new edition of the book and keeping the price very low.

7, Tribune Colony,
Ambala Cantonment-133001.
India.

G.D. Thapar

Preface to the First Edition

High blood pressure is a common disease worldwide, affecting more than 20 per cent of the adult population and over 60 per cent above the age of sixty-five years. With increasing industrialisation and urbanisation of the country and consequent changes in the lifestyle of the people and faster pace of life with increased stress and strain, the incidence of the condition and its complications have shown a disturbing rise.

Hypertension is called a 'silent killer'; silent, because it produces few symptoms but continues doing its damage. Symptoms appear when serious complications affecting vital organs crop up. The proper control of blood pressure and associated disturbances is, therefore, of fundamental importance if such complications have to be prevented.

Control with modern-day therapy is not difficult. While the physician prescribes the medication and makes suitable recommendations for lifestyle changes, the actual control of the condition cannot be achieved without the active and willing cooperation of the patient. The latter needs to be given accurate information about the basic facts of the disease and its complications before he can be expected to make an informed decision to implement those recommendations. This approach can make a real difference in controlling the condition and preventing complications.

It is with this objective that the book is written in simple readable language for the intelligent layman, cutting out all unnecessary terminology and theories.

I also hope that practitioners of medicine will find this book useful as a source of information to which they may refer their hypertensive patients to ensure their full cooperation in the control of their disease.

I am grateful to Dr. Anil Thapar for helping me to write the chapter on hypertension in children and for the suggestions for improvement in the text of the book.

Suggestions and constructive criticism from the readers will be gratefully received.

Ambala Cantt. **G.D. Thapar**

Word of Caution

- The information contained in this book is intended to supplement your doctor's advice and guidance. It is not meant to replace them.
- Do not attempt your own diagnosis.
- Do not try self-treatment; this can be dangerous.
- Diagnosis should always be made by a competent doctor and treatment carried out under his/her professional care.
- This book will help you to carry out the doctor's instructions properly for a better outcome of treatment.

Contents

1

Introduction

What has struck me time and again during my medical practice is the almost complete lack of knowledge and the ignorance of many persons, even the educated lot, about blood pressure and its adverse effects. It is unfortunate because this can lead to only one result: poor control of blood pressure with poor outcome of treatment.

High blood pressure, hypertension as we call it, rarely produces any symptoms. Most patients are blissfully unaware of its existence. Symptoms and complaints arise from its complications, most of which are serious conditions like heart attacks and strokes. The correct time to start treatment is long before the onset of complications. The treatment is given not because the patient is feeling unwell due to high blood pressure, as this is not the case, but is directed towards the prevention of complications and to ensure longevity and a good quality of life without health problems.

God has allocated a life span of four scores and ten to the human species. We owe it to ourselves as well as to our families that we live out this life span in full without creating problems for ourselves and for our near and dear ones. It is also our duty to ensure, as far as possible, that our children do not suffer from this disease when they reach our age.

With increasing industrialisation and urbanisation of the country, many of us are constrained to live a life which can hardly be called natural—a tension-ridden sedentary life, with overuse of auto-vehicles, little physical activity, consumption of junk food and, probably, alcohol. Little wonder then that hypertension is common and is becoming more and more so day by day.

While science has brought material comforts and a fast pace of life and with it hypertension, it has also brought its solutions by way of effective medicines and the understanding of the disease as well as the physiological measures to control it. It is this knowledge, which cannot be imparted by a physician in a single sitting or even in multiple consultations and which every hypertensive person must know, that I wish to share with you in this book. You will know from these pages what havoc this silent disease can cause and why its lifelong control is essential. You will also learn that the disease can be fully controlled, its complications effectively prevented, normal life expectancy restored and a good quality of life looked forward to.

Living in this stressful world of today, you must know how to protect yourself from the adverse effects of hypertension. If God has given us rain, he has also given us the wisdom to use the umbrella. This book is the umbrella against hypertension which I offer to you for your protection. If you use this umbrella, you can be assured of a long and healthy life.

Read on to find out how you can use this umbrella to your best advantage.

2

The Scenario

Let me tell you the true story of a family.

He was born in the year 1900 in a family that had fallen on hard times, having sided with the freedom-fighters against the British in the 1857 uprising. His father was a postmaster in a village getting forty rupees a month. Though forty rupees then was not as insignificant a sum as it is today, it was by no means a comfortable salary. The family lived frugally and somehow made both ends meet. His mother, a small woman of slight build, was fond of smoking 'hukka'. When pregnant with him, any extra food or milk for her was out of question. Not long after his birth, his father died of plague, then raging in India at the turn of the century. The family went into destitution. His grandfather, a petty official of meagre means, brought the family to his house where the orphaned child grew up. After matriculation, he was sent to the nearest college in Lahore. But there was no money, and after a year he had to give up his studies to take up a job as a clerk.

He was intelligent and ambitious, and marriage brought him an equally intelligent and ambitious, though almost illiterate, wife. His mother and a widowed aunt, who had become his responsibility after his grandfather's death, lived with him and his family. He was clear in his mind from the beginning that his children would be educated as professionals. It meant a lot of hard work, stress and sacrifice for both the husband and wife to look after the two widows and bring up five children and educate them according to his standards, by no means small, considering his meagre means and the difficult times of British occupation. He worked hard in the office, earned quick promotions in the face of fierce competition and, by the time he was in his mid-thirties, became reasonably well off.

As comfortable living came with better food and amenities, his blood pressure was found to be rising. He and his family were fond of rich food, highly spiced and salted. Soon, it was found that the wife's blood pressure was also rising. There was no treatment known for hypertension in those days, nor was it known that a rich, high-salt diet caused high blood pressure. So nothing could be done till after 1950 when drugs for hypertension started coming. The doctors then had little experience of using those drugs. Once, when he was in his midfifties, a doctor finding his blood pressure inordinately high gave him two tablets of Adelphane to bring it down. He dropped unconscious. Luckily, nothing worse happened, but the incident showed that the long-standing uncontrolled blood pressure had caused degeneration and damage to the arteries in his brain. He was put on regular treatment for hypertension with whatever drugs were then available. But the damage to the arteries in the brain must have been extensive. While in his sixties, he got the first attack which left him paralysed with Parkinson's disease. With each successive attack, occurring every now and then, he continued deteriorating till the final one four years later which left him in coma for four months before he succumbed to the disease.

His wife, who too had hypertension, also could not have the benefit of antihypertensive drugs. She suffered two major complications of hypertension—a heart attack at the age of 59 and, soon after that, a stroke which left her paralysed, with defects in memory and speech. Though with the control of hypertension with drugs and diet, she lived till the age of eighty-five, but with what quality of life—paralysed for life. The treatment had arrived too late for her. It did prolong her life but could not reverse the damage already done.

The couple did succeed in realising their ambition for their children. All of them were highly educated and became professionals and scientists, and held top positions with the government and universities, but all had hypertension. They were, however, lucky. By the time the disease appeared in them, effective medicines for it had been invented. They have been taking regular treatment. Now in their sixties and seventies, they have remained healthy and none has suffered from any complication of the disease. Their children, the third generation, many well into the fifth decade of their life, are all free of hypertension.

Here ends the story of three generations of the same family—the first who suffered from hypertension and its complications but could not have the benefit of antihypertensive treatment early enough, the second generation who suffered from hypertension but none of its complications because they were lucky to have the benefit of treatment in time, and the third generation who seemed to have escaped the disease altogether. Why? This is an important question which we shall examine in Chapter 8 and find ways of prevention of the disease in Chapter 21.

3

Some Basic Facts

Hypertension is a disease of the blood vessels. For a meaningful discussion on the subject, it is necessary to touch upon a few basic facts about blood vessels, the circulaton of blood and the maintenance of its pressure within the arteries.

Circulation of Blood

Blood circulates throughout the body by means of the heart, which acts as a double muscular pump. Its right side receives blood from the body and pumps it into the lungs for oxygenation. The left side receives oxygenated blood from the lungs and pumps it into the body through the aorta, the main arterial channel of the body.

The arteries carry oxygenated blood from the heart to various parts of the body and the veins bring it back to the heart in unoxygenated state. The blood is thus constantly circulating in the body throughout our lives, because every part of the body has to be supplied with nutrients, water and oxygen without interruption. While oxygen is added to the blood by the lungs, water and nutrients from food are added to it by the alimentary canal, i.e., the intestines.

The arteries are stoutly built tubes made of muscle and elastic tissue. As they approach their destination, i.e., the tissues in various parts of the body, they divide and subdivide into smaller and smaller

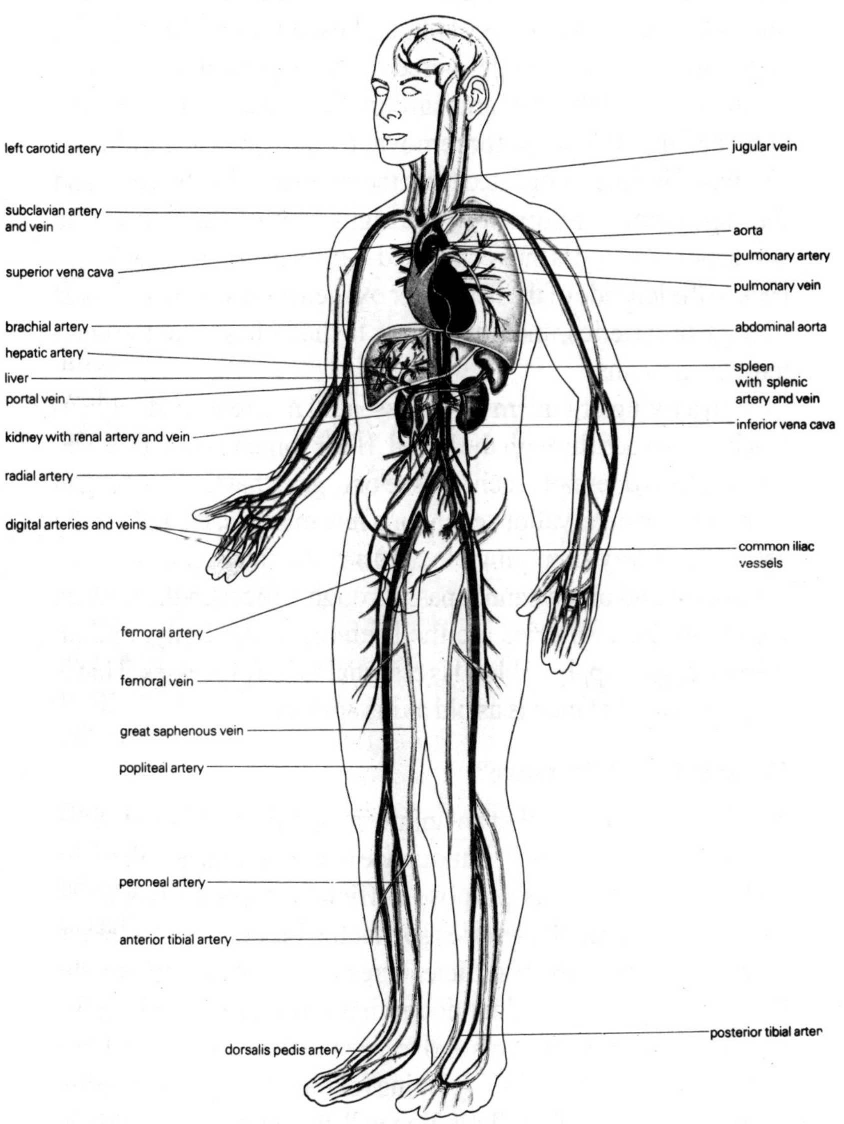

Figure: The circulatory system of the body

branches and finally break up into capillaries. The latter are the finest vessels which are spread out in the tissues. It is through the capillaries that the watery part of blood (plasma) bathes every one of the millions of cells of our bodies. It is here that oxygen, water and nutrients are delivered to the tissues and the waste products of metabolism and carbon dioxide are removed and absorbed into the blood for removal by the lungs and kidneys. The blood is finally collected from the capillaries by the veins and through them is returned to the right side of the heart. The circulation of blood is thus completed—from the heart to the lungs, back to the left side of the heart after oxygenation, on to the tissues through the arteries, and finally back to the right side of the heart through the veins.

In a living organism all the essential nutrients and oxygen reach the tissues through the blood. If for some reason, this life-giving blood does not reach a tissue or organ, that tissue or organ dies. Oxygen deprivation, even for a few minutes, is fatal for the cells. If an artery supplying blood to a particular organ becomes obstructed and blood cannot pass through it to reach the tissues, the organ dies. Arteries are the lifelines of the body, and an uninterrupted supply of blood is essential to life processes. That is why it is said that man is as old as his arteries.

What is Blood Pressure?

You have seen above that an uninterrupted flow of blood in the blood vessels is of utmost importance to the life and health of the body tissues. For this purpose sufficient pressure has to be maintained within the arteries so that the blood is able to reach every part of the body. If sufficient pressure is not maintained, the flow of blood may so slow down that it is unable to reach the tissues and supply nutrients and oxygen to them. Slowing down may also lead to thrombosis (clotting) of blood within the arteries, causing obstruction to its flow. You will, therefore, appreciate that a certain minimum pressure of blood within the arteries is essential for maintaining normal life. This pressure of blood within the arteries is called blood pressure.

How is Blood Pressure Maintained?

Blood pressure is maintained by the force of the pumping action of the heart and by the tone or constriction of the small peripheral arteries. I will illustrate this by a simple experiment. Attach a rubber tubing to a rubber bladder, full of water. The harder you press the bladder, the greater will be the pressure with which the water will flow out of the tube. Also, if you constrict or pinch the end of the rubber tubing with your fingers, the pressure of the flow of water will increase even though you have not increased the force of compression on the bladder. In a similar manner, the blood pressure depends upon the force of the heartbeat as well as the tone of the peripheral blood vessels. If you run or make strenuous physical effort, your heart beats faster and with greater force, raising the blood pressure. If the tone of the peripheral blood vessels increases or they constrict due to, say, cold in winter, the blood pressure rises, even though force of contraction of the heart has remained unchanged. The greater the tone of the blood vessels, the higher is the blood pressure. This is precisely what happens in hypertension. The tone of the small perpheral arteries is inordinately increased, raising the blood pressure all over the arterial tree. The elevated blood pressure day in and day out produces its deleterious effects on the arteries and the heart. How these effects on the arteries are produced, what damage they inflict on the vital organs, and how you can protect yourself from these ill-effects are what you will learn from the subsequent pages.

4

How to Measure Blood Pressure

Members of hypertensive families should learn and practise the use of the blood pressure instrument and should be able to measure and record blood pressure. This is not difficult.

Types of Instruments

Three types of blood pressure instruments are in user :

1. Mercury sphygmomanometer
2. Dial (spring) Type
3. Electronic

The cheapest and most accurate instrument is the mercury sphygmomanometer. It can become inaccurate only if some mercury leaks out. Accuracy can be ensured simply by checking the mercury level before inflating: it should be at zero. If there is a leakage, get it corrected before use.

The spring type instruments are liable to give erroneous readings as the tension of the spring wears out in course of time. They need to be calibrated with a mercury instrument now and then.

The electronic instruments are easy to use, do not need a stethoscope and can, therefore, be used for self-measurement of blood pressure. But all these advantages are offset by the fact that they sometimes give erroneous readings and can be the cause of a false alarm and consequent wrong treatment. Moreover, they are expensive.

It is recommended that you buy a good mercury type instrument. Buy one with an ISI mark. Buy a reasonably good stethoscope; an expensive fancy stethoscope is not required for this purpose.

Method

- The patient should be sitting or lying at ease.
- The instrument should be placed at your eye level.
- All clothing from the arm should be removed.
- The cuff (standard width for adults is 12.5 cm) should be applied closely to the arm, about 1 inch above the elbow, with the rubber bladder (inside the cuff) on the inner side of the arm. A narrower cuff may record falsely high pressures.
- Place the stethoscope lightly over the artery in the elbow. (It lies at the junction of the middle-third and inner-third of elbow.)
- Inflate the rubber bulb; the mercury will rise in the glass tube.
- You will start hearing the sound of the pulse beat. Go on inflating till the sound disappears and the mercury goes at least 30 mm above the level of the disappearance of the sound.
- The pressure in the cuff is gradually lowered by opening the pressure release valve. The mercury will start falling. The first sound you hear is the systolic pressure. Continue to lower the pressure in the cuff till the sound becomes suddenly faint or disappears. This is the diastolic pressure.
- The blood pressure readings are expressed as:
  Systolic pressure 140 mm Hg; Diastolic pressure 86 mm Hg; or simply as 140/86.
- It is better to take three readings and accept the average.
- After you have practised the procedure, get a few readings checked by your doctor.

- Record the readings in a diary kept for the purpose along with the date and time of the readings.
- The diary should be shown to your doctor at regular intervals, or earlier if the blood pressure goes out of control.

The best time to measure blood pressure is in the morning before breakfast after resting for fifteen minutes.

5

Normal and Abnormal Blood Pressure

What is Normal Blood Pressure?

It is not easy to define normal blood pressure because there are fairly wide variations from person to person and from time to time in the same person.

Currently, 130/80 is considered normal BP and 140/90 upper limit of normal blood pressure at rest in the fourth decade of life. Somewhat lower figures have to be accepted as the upper limit of normal blood pressure in younger individuals.

The figure of 140/90 has been so determined on the basis of worldwide records which show that blood pressure above this figure tends to cause damage to the arteries of important organs like the heart, brain, eyes and kidneys.

Optimal blood pressure, as distinct from upper normal, is considered to be 120/80 in adults.

Changes in Blood Pressure with Age

Normally, the upper range of blood pressure rises with age. The upper limit of normal blood pressure at different ages is given below:

Age	Upper limit of normal blood pressure
1 year	100/70
13 years	120/80
18 years	130/85
35 years	140/90

Abnormal Blood Pressure

Blood pressure may be abnormal if it is too high (hypertension), or too low (hypotension).

Hypertension

The blood pressure rises physiologically above the resting level after work or exercise, or during fever and excitement. This is not hypertension. Raised blood pressure is called hypertension if at rest it is found to be higher than 140/90 on three separate occasions.

Degree of Hypertension

Currently, hypertension is categorised on the basis of its severity as under:-

130/80 or lower	Normal
130/80 to 140/90	Upper range of normal; recheck 6 monthly
140/90 to 160/100	Mild hypertension; recheck to confirm
160/100 to 180/110	Moderate hypertension
Above 180/110	Severe hypertension

Above 200/120 and/or vital organ involvement	Accelerated hypertension; emergency

The patient's visit to the doctor tends to cause some degree of excitement, with consequent rise of blood pressure in some persons (White coat reaction). If this is not taken into account, overdiagnosis of the disease is likely in border-line and mild cases. For this reason, WHO recommends that in every mild or borderline case monthly readings should be taken for a few months to allow this reaction to wear off, so that unnecessary treatment, which is life-long, is not started on inadequate grounds.

Systolic Hypertension

Sometimes only the systolic pressure rises and if found to be consistently above 150 mm, but the diastolic pressure remains below 90 mm. This is called systolic hypertension. These patients may also run the risk of developing complications depending upon the degree of their blood pressure.

It is important to emphasise that high blood pressure may produce few symptoms and the patient may be unaware of its existence till serious complications occur. It is not at all unusual for doctors to come across patients with very high blood pressure, even above 200/120, and the patients with very high blood pressure, even above 200/120, and the patients not feeling anything amiss. Hypertension is a silent killer. Therefore, one should never depend upon one's feelings to judge the level of blood pressure; the only rational method is a check with the BP instrument.

Low Blood Pressure (Hypotension)

Many young people come to the doctor complaining of 'low blood pressure'. They may have some indefinite symptoms of fatigue or general debility, but may otherwise be in good health. It may be stated for their information that it is perfectly normal to have BP readings of 110/70 or even 100/70. In effect, habitually low blood pressure, not caused by any disease process, is a blessing. It is a different matter, however, if the blood pressure falls as a result of some disease, e.g., a heart attack or bleeding. It may then be a matter of concern and urgent treatment may be required for the causative condition.

6

Causes of High Blood Pressure

In the vast majority (almost 90 to 95 per cent) of cases of hypertension the cause is unknown. This is called 'essential hypertension'. There is no disease to account for the elevated blood pressure, but it is usually associated with certain metabolic abnormalities, which are not its cause but its accompaniments. They all need to be looked for and taken care of by your doctor for a satisfactory outcome of the treatment. For this reason, this group is now referred to as the 'hypertension syndrome' (Chapter 7). Since this essential hypertension accounts for the vast majority of cases of hypertension, most of the discussion that follows relates to this condition.

The other, minority group comprising only 5-10 per cent of the cases, has some underlying disease as its cause and is, therefore, called 'secondary hypertension'. The causes are diverse—inflammatory kidney disease (nephritis), inborn abnormalities of the aorta or urinary tract, diseases of hormone glands, etc. Some hormone preparations like contraceptive pills and corticosteroid preparations, and some nasal drops for colds can raise the blood pressure temporarily.

Hypertension occurring before the age of 30 is usually secondary to some other disease. The latter may be a curable condition. If so, as in the case of surgical operation for inborn abnormality of aorta, the treatment may not only cure the abnormality but also the hypertension.

7

The Hypertension Syndrome

Not very long ago, hypertension was considered to be just elevated blood pressure, and it was thought that if it was lowered and maintained at near-normal levels, all would be well.

But, all has not been well. Since the introduction of Reserpine, the first drug to lower blood pressure, in 1950, more and more new and effective drugs have been introduced. Over the last four decades we have collected a wealth of experience and data from large-scale clinical trials all over the world. Lowering the blood pressure has markedly reduced the incidence of brain haemorrhage and left heart failure (cardiac asthma), but the incidence of heart attacks has not been brought down impressively.

It is now realised that hypertension is not merely elevated blood pressure, though it is a very important component of the disease. It is a syndrome or collection of certain metabolic abnormalities in addition to high blood pressure. These abnormalities may be acquired through heredity or acquired early in life (see next chapter). Some or many of them may coexist with the raised blood pressure. They are:

- Sensitisation to sodium (common salt). It is directly responsible for raising the blood pressure.
- Abnormalities of potassium, as also calcium and magnesium transport in the cells; their deficiency and imbalance with

sodium is believed to elevate the blood pressure.

- Abnormalities of fat metabolism: lipids or fats circulate in the blood in the form of cholesterol and neutral fats (triglycerides). Cholesterol is in two forms: LDL-cholesterol which is damaging to the arteries and HDL-cholesterol which is beneficial and protective. In hypertension, total cholesterol and LDL-cholesterol may be high and HDL-cholesterol low. Triglycerides also may be high.
- Abnormalities of sugar metabolism; the body may lose sensitivity to insulin, which causes rise of blood sugar and diabetes.
- Abnormalities of the clotting mechanism may be responsible for easy coagulability of blood within the arteries, precipitating strokes and heart attacks.
- Obesity.
- Blood uric acid may be raised and may cause gout.

These abnormalities raise the blood pressure and, as you will see later, are responsible for arterial damage and blockage with fatty deposits, the ultimate cause of damage to vital organs like the heart and brain.

You will appreciate that while in any hypertensive patient it is important to lower the blood pressure and maintain it at near normal levels, this alone is not enough. For the optimum control and prevention of complications, your doctor will investigate you for these abnormalities and take care of those found in you.

8

Development of Hypertension

Traditionally, certain genetic and constitutional factors (e.g., Type A personality) are considered to be responsible for the rise of blood pressure in some individuals, and certain environmental factors to aggravate it.

Early Origin of Hypertension

While the importance of the aforementioned factors cannot be minimised, the focus of attention has recently shifted to factors in intrauterine life and early infancy. It is now believed that early factors may profoundly affect the subsequent development of hypertension in later life, and that the origin of hypertension and cardiovascular disease is 'programmed' during the period of rapid growth in early life. The term 'programming' is used for the long-term changes in the body's structure, physiology and metabolism brought about by environmental influences acting at critical stages of life within the womb and immediately after.

Maternal malnutrition, anaemia and heavy smoking during pregnancy are considered to have an important adverse influence on programming by effecting failure of proper maturation of tissues during critical periods of growth. This failure of proper maturation is to some extent irrecoverable, and in course of time causes hypertension and cardiovascular disease.

Interesting studies have been reported from Preston. They have shown that babies, who have a small head size, a low birth weight and are thin in relation to their gestational age (i.e., these characteristics are not due to premature birth but to growth retardation within the womb), tend as adults to develop hypertension, disordered fat and sugar metabolism and run a higher risk of heart attacks and strokes. Many researchers have suggested that these changes reflect non-maturation of certain tissues and programme for hypertension and cardiovascular disease in later life.

Operation of Environmental Factors

After the body has been so programmed, all appears to be well for a number of decades, though the blood pressure of the children destined to become hypertensive may be higher than the average blood pressure of other children of the same age. When these children grow to middle age, their blood pressure starts rising under the influence of the environmental factors which go with affluence.

The prime environmental factors which have been indentified are:

- excess salt
- inadequate potassium (also calcium and magnesium)
- stress and competition
- excess calories, causing obesity
- excess alcohol

Metabolic abnormalities, affecting fat and sugar metabolism may appear around the same time as high blood pressure. They are also accentuated by factors which go with affluence. They are:

- excess of animal fat
- smoking
- lack of exercise

- sedentary habits
- overuse of auto-vehicles and physical inactivity

It is interesting to observe from the above discussion that a combination of factors associated with early adversity and later affluence are considered responsible for high blood pressure, its associated metabolic abnormalities and adverse effects. Maternal health and nutrition and avoidance of smoking by the pregnant lady are of utmost importance so as to provide a healthy environment to the unborn child, and thus prevent hypertension and its complications in later life.

All the environmental factors enumerated above are modifiable. In Chapter 13, we shall examine how best we can modify them to our best advantage.

9

Development of Adverse Effects

Hypertension is a biting dog which seldom barks. Silently, imperceptibly and without producing symptoms, it goes on inflicting damage on the vital organs. The adverse effects are related to two phenomena—the degeneration and blockage of the arteries, and the mechanical effects of the high pressure of blood obtaining in the arterial tree.

Blockage of Arteries

Arteries are the lifelines of the body through which life-giving blood carrying oxygen, water and nutrients is supplied to every part of the body. By a slow and steady process of degeneration, hypertension produces a thickening of the arterial wall and deposits of fatty material (cholesterol) on the walls of the arteries. These deposits, which are called atheroma, obstruct the flow of blood in the affected arteries. They occur in the major arteries supplying blood to the heart, brain, kidneys, legs, etc. and even in the mother of all arteries, the aorta. Wherever the arteries are clogged beyond a critical degree, the blood supply to that part is obstructed and symptoms relevant to that part are produced. If in the heart, angina appears; if in the brain, transient ischaemic attacks (temporary paralysis) may appear. If blood clots (thrombosis) on top of the atheroma, blood supply may be completely cut off, and a heart attack or stroke may be produced. The manifestation, therefore, depends upon the site and degree of obstruction. You will, therefore, appreciate that many apparently diverse diseases are produced by the obstruction in the arteries. The health of the arteries is of utmost importance. Man is as old as his arteries.

Deposition of cholesterol on the arterial wall and production of atheroma do not occur in a day; it is a gradual process extending over years. High blood pressure aided and abetted by the associated metabolic abnormalities of high blood cholesterol, especially LDL-cholesterol, high blood sugar (diabetes), unhealthy lifestyle, stress, heavy smoking, excess of alcohol, lack of exercise and obesity results in the clogging of the arteries. You will, therefore, realise that while lowering the elevated blood pressure is important, that alone is not enough without taking care of the other risk factors which may be operating in a particular case. However, it needs to be clarified that in a particular patient of hypertension all the risk factors and metabolic disturbances need not be present but only some and they may have to be dug out by laboratory investigations.

Mechanical Effects of Hypertension

There are other ways in which high blood pressure affects the arteries. If there is a rise of pressure to very high levels, the arteries may be unable to withstand it and may burst causing haemorrhage.

Hypertension may affect the heart directly by its pressure effects. The left ventricle of the heart, the principal pumping chamber, has to work against the resistance of high blood pressure day in and day out. It compensates by hypertrophy and enlargement of its muscle mass. But there is a limit to this compensation. When this limit is crossed, the heart fails in its function as a pump; left ventricular failure results with severe difficulty of breathing (cardiac asthma).

By acting on the fine blood vessels of the kidneys and retina of the eyes, hypertension causes their degeneration which adversely affects the health and function of these organs. This effect is more likely to occur if diabetes is present in addition to hypertension.

In the following pages we shall discuss in some detail the disease conditions produced by hypertension to help you to recognise them and take timely action, if and when an occasion arises.

10

Hypertension-related Diseases

In this chapter we shall take a closer look at the specific disease conditions caused by hypertension, so that you are able to recognise them, if any of them occurs, and take timely action. The organs which are targeted for damage are the heart, brain, kidneys, eyes and legs. The diseases are, therefore, related to these organs; the commonest and most important being heart attacks and strokes.

(I) ANGINA AND HEART ATTACKS

The commonest complication of hypertension is ischaemic heart disease, which manifests as angina pectoris (angina for short) and heart attacks. As we have seen in the previous chapter, it is caused by obstructing fatty deposits of cholesterol on the wall of the coronary arteries which supply blood to the heart. These cholesterol deposits, called atheroma, cause narrowing of lumen of the artery leading to insufficient blood supply (ischaemia) to a segment of the heart. That is why the disease is called by the generic names of ischaemic heart disease (IHD) and coronary artery disease (CAD) Both these terms are synonymous with the disease which manifests as angina and heart attacks.

Angina Pectoris

Angina is a heart pain of short duration lasting not more than twenty minutes. It is a cry of the heart muscle due to a temporary imbalance between demand and supply of oxygen. It is caused by partial obstruction of a coronary artery by cholesterol deposits, so that the blood supply to a segment of the heart muscle, sufficient while at rest, becomes insufficient when the work of the heart is increased due to exertion.

Recognition of Angina

Angina can be recognised by its symptoms—the character of the pain and its radiation. The pain is constricting, squeezing or choking, or as if a heavy weight has been placed on the chest. Some patients experience a severe burning pain in the pit of the stomach or behind the lower end of the breast bone and insist that the pain is due to dyspepsia. The pain is invariably situated in the central portion of the front of the chest in the region of the lower portion of the breast bone. Although the heart lies more to the left, the pain is rarely felt there. The pain may radiate to the left shoulder and arm, right shoulder and arm or both, to the neck or lower jaw, or directly to the back into the area between the shoulder blades. Sometimes, no pain may be felt in the chest but only in one of the sites of radiation, i.e., the shoulder, arm, neck, jaw or even the pit of the stomach. The patient may feel very anxious.

The pain lasts for a few minutes, not more than twenty. It is related to physical effort like brisk walking, going uphill or climbing stairs, or after emotional outbursts, anger or fright or sexual activity. There is, however, a severe form of angina called unstable angina, in which the pain may appear during rest, may last for more than twenty minutes and may recur often. Usually these cases end up in a heart attack, i.e., myocardial infarction.

The anginal pain is relieved by discontinuing the exertion and by nitroglycerine (Angised). After the pain is relieved, the patient may feel well enough to resume his activity.

Confirmatory or corroborative evidence is sought in the electrocardiogram (ECG). Taken at rest, the ECG may be within normal limits. The patient is then made to exercise on a two-step

(Master's) stool, stationary cycle or a treadmill, and the ECG repeated to check if changes due to ischaemia appear. He is investigated for the presence of risk factors like diabetes, high blood cholesterol, etc. (Chapter 11), so that they can be suitably dealt with.

Since the presence of angina indicates the existence of ischaemic heart disease and, therefore, an increased proneness to heart attacks, the treatment is directed not only towards alleviation of the symptoms with antianginal drugs (nitrates like sorbitrate and angised, betablocking drugs like Inderal, calcium channel blocking drugs like Diltiazem, etc.), but also to prevent heart attacks. In this context, changes in lifestyle such as giving up smoking, reduction of weight, control of diabetes and hypertension and the use of vegetable oil as cooking medium are called for. The reader is strongly advised to adopt the lifestyle suggested in Chapter 20, which incorporates all these and many more points important to the hypertensive patient's health. By way of drugs, Aspirin in a dose of 50-100 mg daily along with antioxidant vitamins A, C and E is all that is necessary to prevent heart attacks. It is important to take aspirin in an enteric coated form like ASA-50, or in a soluble form like Colsprin-100 which should be dissolved in a glass of water. Take it immediately after meals. These precautions are necessary to prevent injury to the delicate lining of the stomach by aspirin which is to be taken daily indefinitely.

Myocardial Infarction (Heart Attack)

Myocardial infarction results from necrosis and death of a segment of the heart muscle. This occurs when an obstruction in a coronary artery becomes complete due to the clotting of blood on a patch of atheroma on the arterial wall, cutting off the blood supply to that segment of the heart muscle.

Recognition of Heart Attack

In a heart attack, the characteristic nature of the pain and its radiation are no different from those in angina pectoris, but it is usually more severe and much more prolonged; it may last for hours and keep recurring for days. There are other symptoms too—profound weakness, profuse cold sweats, palpitations, sometimes difficulty in breathing and there may be a deathly pallor. However, not all symptoms may be present in a particular patient.

The severity of the pain is no index of the severity of the attack. Some patients may have only a little pain or even no pain at all, but only sudden profound weakness with cold sweats and pallor. Any middle-aged or older person having these indefinite symptoms will have to be carefully observed and investigated by a physician for possible myocardial infarction.

Dangers Faced by the Patient

The dangers arise from the following complications:

- disturbances of the heart rhythm causing irregular heart action;
- fall of blood pressure which may be precipitate or rapid;
- failure of the pumping function of the heart, especially of the left ventricle, causing severe difficulty in breathing, gasping for air, cough and frothy bloodstained sputum (left ventricular failure or cardiac asthma);
- clotting of blood in the leg veins, the clot may break loose and go to the lungs; and
- stroke and paralysis.

These complications are mentioned here merely for the information of the reader. It is, of course, the job of the attending physician to constantly watch out for them, prevent them as far as possible and treat them if and when they occur.

Confirmation of the attack is made by the physician with the help of an ECG and other laboratory investigations. It is important to emphasise the fact that in the first few hours or even days the ECG may show little or only a slight deviation from the normal, yet the patient would need all the care necessary for a seriously ill person. Serial ECGs and laboratory investigations are usually necessary not only to confirm the diagnosis but also to monitor the progress of the case.

Differentiation between Angina and Heart Attack

Any single attack of angina is usually not dangerous to life, and can and should be treated by the patient himself with nitroglycerine (Angised), prescribed by his doctor. But since the character and location of the pain of angina and heart attack are the same, it is important for the patient or his/her relatives to recognise when the attack of pain is no longer simple angina but is a heart attack, so that immediate action can be taken. This can be done by observing certain important points.

Any heart pain which

- has not subsided in twenty minutes after rest;
- has not responded to the usual dose of nitroglycerine (or sorbitrate) given twice or thrice under the tongue;
- continues to recur;
- is accompanied by:
  - –profound weakness
  - –cold sweats
  - –palpitations
  - –irregular pulse (if you can make out)
  - –difficulty in breathing

is likely to be an attack of myocardial infarction and needs urgent cardiac care, usually in an intensive coronary care unit. If there is any doubt, a physician must be consulted without loss of time, to decide whether or not such care is necessary.

Importance of Early Recognition of Heart Attack

It is of extreme importance to recognise the symptoms of a heart attack at the earliest possible moment and place the patient under expert cardiological care, because the first few hours are most crucial when serious complications are a common occurrence; secondly, there are therapies which are effective only if administered in the first four to six hours of the attack, the earlier the better, e.g., thrombolytic therapy with streptokinase or urokinase.

Apart from investigating for the attack, the patient is investigated for the presence or absence of risk factors as in the case of angina, so that his lifestyle may be suitably altered, and other preventive measures instituted to avoid future attacks.

Role of Surgery in IHD

Coronary bypass surgery, which means bypassing the obstruction in the coronary artery, is necessary only in those cases of angina where symptoms of anginal pain are severe and remain unrelieved by medical treatment or if the angina is so prolonged and unstable that there is imminent danger or myocardial infarction.

Coronary angiography, i.e., X-rays of the coronary arteries after injecting contrast medium is done to find out where exactly thc obstruction lies, before the patient can be evaluated for surgery. It may be added here that coronary angiography is required only for those cases where surgery is envisaged. It is neither necessary nor desirable if no operation is contemplated, because it does not help improve the medical treatment.

An attempt can also be made to remove the obstruction in the coronary artery by the semi-surgical technique of coronary angioplasty. In this the atheroma is pressed down by a small balloon passed through a catheter into the coronary artery. The problem, however, is that the rate of reocclusion is high. For this procedure also coronary angiography is essential.

It may be pointed out that the above procedures are useful steps in the total care of the coronary patient, but they are not a panacea for ischaemic heart disease. They cannot take the place of preventive measures, the importance of which cannot be overemphasised. These measures must form part of the lifestyle of every hypertensive patient (chapter 21), whether or not he has ischaemic heart disease.

(II) CARDIAC ASTHMA

Apart from IHD, the heart can be affected directly by the mechanical effects of high blood pressure. The left ventricle, the principal pumping chamber of the heart, has to push blood against high pressure obtaining in the arteries. As a compensation for the increasing work, the muscle mass of the ventricle goes on increasing. But there is a limit to this compensation. Ultimately it fails in its pumping function (left ventricular failure). Since it is unable to pump out all the blood received from the lungs, a backlog of blood results in the lungs. Due to the high pressure of blood in the lungs, the watery part of the blood is forced out into the spongy spaces in the lungs. The patient becomes severely breathless and has air hunger and cough. This is cardiac asthma, and is a very serious condition, very different from the ordinary asthma. An acute and sudden rise of untreated and uncontrolled blood pressure can precipitate this condition. It is a medical emergency and needs to be treated in the ICCU.

(III) BRAIN THROMBOSIS

One of the serious and common complications of hypertension is thrombotic stroke or cerebral thrombosis. It is less common than heart attacks and, like the latter, is caused by the obstructive process of atheroma formation in an artery of the brain and a blood clot forming over it. Since the blood supply to the affected area is cut off, that area of the brain dies. The symptoms would depend upon the area affected. Different areas of the brain control different functions, e.g., we have areas controlling body movements, sensations of touch, pain and temperature, hearing, speech, sight, ideation, memory, emotions, etc. Each of the two hemispheres of the brain controls opposite side of the body. The speech centre is located on the left side in right-handed individuals and on the right side in the left-handed. If the dominant side is involved in the paralysis (hemiplegia), speech may also be affected. However, speech defects alone can arise if only the speech area is involved. When hemiplegia occurs there is a large area of the brain surrounding the necrosed brain tissue which is not dead but under the stress of oedema (swelling) and deficient blood supply. As this area recovers, the patient shows improvement. Therefore, after a few months of an attack of complete hemiplegia the patient may recover enough to be able to walk about with a limp. His speech and memory, if affected, may also return in part. The improvement may be quite remarkable in some patients. The patients may continue to progress for almost eighteen months or so.

If the patient is unable to speak or his speech is unintelligible, it does not necessarily mean that he cannot understand what you may be talking. In fact, many patients can understand perfectly well, and can become very agitated and disturbed if something inappropriate is spoken in their hearing. Hence the relatives and friends have to be cautious while talking lest they unintentionally hurt the patient's feelings.

Minor Strokes

Sometimes minor strokes occur, which may cause only subtle changes in the person's behaviour, personality, speech, memory or intellect, perceptible only to people close to the person like the spouse or children. These minor strokes are due to small clots in the arteries of the brain.

Transient Ischaemic Attacks

There may be transient ischaemic attacks (TIA) which may cause paralysis or affect the speech or some other function of the brain. These are short-lived, last a few hours or days and then disappear completely. These attacks are due to insufficient blood supply and are analogous to angina pectoris, i.e., heart pain of short duration. Unless preventive measures are taken, these attacks may end up in a major attack and paralysis.

Risk Factors and Their Prevention

Hypertension is the most well-defined risk factor for strokes. The other risk factors, many of which may coexist with high blood pressure, are high blood cholesterol, diabetes, obesity, lack of physical activity and exercise, cigarette smoking, etc. They are the same as for IHD, though their role has not yet been fully defined. In the present state of knowledge, all the precautions necessary against heart attacks, control of hypertension in particular, should be considered useful to prevent thrombotic strokes.

Just as the sudden rise of blood pressure cannot be tolerated by old and degenerated arteries, sudden and/or excessive fall of blood pressure due to any cause, including an overdose of medication for hypertension, can precipitate cerebral thrombosis by slowing down blood circulation in the brain and should, therefore, be avoided.

(IV) BRAIN HAEMORRHAGE

Brain haemorrhage or haemorrhagic stroke is caused by the rupture of an artery in the brain, which causes interruption of blood supply as well as bleeding into the brain substance. The effect is the destruction of the latter. As in thrombosis, the symptoms depend upon the area involved, but they are more sudden, more severe and advance more quickly. The patient may become unconscious (coma) and the outcome is more gloomy.

The usual cause of cerebral haemorrhage is the sudden rise of blood pressure to very high levels, above 200 mm systolic or 130 mm diastolic. Old and degenerated arteries are unable to withstand such high pressures and burst. In young pregnant women, sometimes toxaemia of pregnancy (Chapter 17) occurs with the rise of blood pressure. In such cases even lower figures like 170/110 can be dangerous and cause cerebral haemorrhage.

Recent research has pointed out that a dangerous synergism exists between high blood pressure and smoking, so much so that hypertensive heavy smokers (more than 20 cigarettes per day) are at 20 times the risk of stroke than non-smokers with normal blood pressure. This high risk can be brought down substantially in two years, and to the level of non-smokers in five years by stopping smoking and controlling the blood pressure. See Chapter 13 (ix) also.

Sudden rises of blood pressure to dangerous levels usually occur in hypertensive patients whose blood pressure is either uncontrolled or poorly controlled. At the cost of repetition, I must stress that even very high levels of blood pressure may not produce any symptoms. A patient may be unaware of his/her high blood pressure, and may become aware of it only when serious symptoms of a complication make their appearance. Proper control of your blood pressure under the watchful eye of your physician cannot be overemphasised.

(V) INTERMITTENT CLAUDICATION

Arterial obstruction by fatty deposits (atheroma) is not confined to the arteries of the heart and brain; it is a general disease of the arteries and occurs in the aorta and its larger branches, including those going to the lower limbs. By the age of sixty, most people can be presumed to have atheromatous lesion spread over their arterial tree. Such lesions may be profound in those suffering from uncontrolled high blood pressure and/or diabetes, and especially those who have an unhealthy lifestyle marked by excessive smoking and drinking, lack of physical activity and obesity.

The lesions in the aorta may remain symptomless unless they produce an obstruction at critical points like the bifurcation of the aorta, i.e., where it divides into its two main branches, one for each leg. The lesions in the arteries in the legs are much less likely to give trouble than the coronary artery lesions. When one of them does, it many cause ischaemic pain in the calf muscles while walking. The pain is relieved by rest. This is called 'intermittent claudication'. In rare cases, clotting of blood may occur in the diseased artery, blocking it completely and cutting off the blood supply to the part of the leg below the obstruction. The result is gangrene.

Blockage higher up at the bifurcation of the aorta causes claudication to occur in the buttocks and thighs along with impotence in the case of males.

(VI) COMPLICATIONS OF ACCELERATED (MALIGNANT) HYPERTENSION

If hypertension remains untreated or uncontrolled, sometimes there is a rapid rise of blood pressure to above 130 mm diastolic, and a rapid downhill course with consequent damage to vital organs in a brief period of time.

Unremitted and uncontrolled hypertension has a devastating effect on the minute blood vessels of the kidneys and eyes, particularly if diabetes is also present. Adverse changes in the eyes and damage to the kidneys occur because of disturbances of blood flow in these organs. The patient is restless, confused, has blurred vision, headache, nausea and vomiting.

Extremely high blood pressure may cause the left ventricle of the heart to fail and cause severe difficulty in breathing. Oedema (swelling) of the brain may occur which causes its dysfunction (encephalopathy) with signs of reversible paralysis.

Accelerated hypertension is an extreme emergency and the patient needs to be treated in an intensive care unit. The blood pressure needs to be carefully brought down to below 100 mm diastolic and kept at that level, and suitable treatment gives early enough to prevent complications. If diabetes coexists, its proper control is equally important.

It must be mentioned that kidney damage is irreversible, but it occurs only in a small minority of patients. It can largely be prevented by proper treatment and control of hypertension and of diabetes, if it coexists. Similarly, the eyes can be protected from adverse effects of the disease by its effective control.

(VII) DIABETES

Diabetes mellitus, that is the full name, is a common condition. Not infrequently it accompanies hypertension, and, when present, adds its own weight as a serious risk factor for the heart and blood vessels, brain, eyes and kidneys. It has many other adverse effects too.

It is a condition in which the sugar metabolism of the body is deranged. In normal people the sugar (glucose), to which all carbohydrates we eat are broken down by the body, is metabolised in the muscles and other tissues with the help of insulin, a hormone produced by a gland called the pancreas. In diabetes, there is either a deficiency of insulin production or blockage of its action and tissues become insensitive to it. The result is that the tissues are unable to metabolise the sugar to get their energy requirement, and the sugar accumulates in the blood. Glucose levels in the blood rise and when they go up to 180 mg% or higher, sugar starts leaking into the urine.

Derangement of sugar metabolism disturbs the rest of the body metabolism too, including lipid (fat) metabolism. Blood cholesterol and LDL-cholesterol rise, which hasten the development of fatty deposits in the arteries with increased and early susceptibility to heart attacks and strokes.

The high level of sugar in the blood and tissues leads to infections such as boils and carbuncles, as well as chronic diseases like tuberculosis. Diabetes can adversely affect many organs, including the eyes and kidneys. Untreated severe diabetes may cause coma and untimely death.

Diabetes cannot be radically cured in the present state of knowledge, but it can be well controlled by a proper diet (see Appendix I), and if necessary, by injections of insulin or oral antidiabetic drugs. To a large extent proper control of diabetes prevents complications. Many complications such as diabetic coma or infections can be completely prevented; the early onset of ischaemic heart disease or strokes may also be prevented.

If you are hypertensive with diabetes, you must maintain proper restrictions on your diet. Like hypertension, control of diabetes is a lifelong process. Half-hearted measures do not work. The control should be a proper one under the directions of your physician, so as to ensure prevention of complications.

11

Laboratory Investigations

You may ask a very logical question: Why are laboratory investigations necessary for hypertension when a diagnosis of the disease is simply made with the help of a blood pressure instrument? Yes, the diagnosis that high blood pressure exists is simple enough but it is important to find out:

- If there are any associated abnormalities in the metabolism of lipids (fats), sugar or uric acid, which would be additional risk factors for the heart and other vital organs. After all, the treatment of hypertension is directed to one single goal—the prevention of complications.
- If any damage has occurred to the target organs and if so, to what extent, so that measures can be taken to halt that damage and undo it to whatever extent possible.
- If there is any underlying disease present, so that corrective action can be taken for the causative condition.

Basic Laboratory Tests

These laboratory tests are done in all cases, whether of the essential variety or secondary to some other disease.

(1) *Urine examination* is done for sugar, protein and microscopy to find evidence, if any, of infection or damage to the kidneys.

(2) *Urine culture and sensitivity* is done if pus cells are found in the urine on routine examination.

(3) *Blood urea and serum creatinine* level is raised if there is kidney damage.

Blood urea	Normal	20-40 mg%
Serum creatinine	Normal	less than 1.5 mg%

(4) *Blood lipids (fats)* are implicated in the formation of fatty deposits (atheroma) in the arteries (Chapter 9) and thus cause heart attack and stroke. Abnormal lipid profile commonly occurs in hypertensive patients as an accompaniment of the disease or sometimes as a result of unsuitable therapy. Two types of lipids are involved, cholesterol and neutral fats called triglycerides. Cholesterol is the fatty substance that gets deposited in the arterial wall to form the atheroma. A high intake of cholesterol containing foods (eggs, organ meat, butter, ghee) keeps the blood cholesterol high and, over the years, it gets deposited in the arterial wall.

Blood cholesterol	Normal	150-220 mg%
	Borderline	220-250 mg%
	High	above 250 mg%

There are two types of cholesterol: LDL-cholesterol, which tends to form atheroma, and HDL-cholesterol, which is protective and beneficial.

HDL-cholesterol	Normal	40-90 mg% (but not less than 25% of total cholesterol)

The role of triglycerides in the causation of atheroma is not yet clear.

Triglycerides	Normal	35-150 mg%
	Borderline	150-190 mg%
	High	above 190 mg%

(5) *Blood sugar* estimation is done to detect the presence of diabetes which, even if mild, worsens the prognosis of hypertension. Many borderline or mild cases remain

undetected for the simple reason that only the urine specimen before breakfast is examined for sugar when blood sugar is lower, the last meal having been taken twelve hours earlier the previous night. Since even mild diabetes continues doing its damage, it is important to ensure by blood sugar estimation that no case of diabetes goes undetected.

Blood sugar levels:

All hypertensive should have their blood sugar checked at least once a year.

Fasting	Normal	80-100mg%
	Impaired fasting glucose	100-110mg%
	Diabetes	above 110mg% on two separate days
Two hours after meals	Normal upto 130	120-140mg%
	Impaired glucose tolerance	130-180mg%
	Diabetes	above 180mg% on two separate occasions

(6) *Blood uric acid,* when high, causes gout. It is also known that the incidence of heart attacks is higher in such cases than in the general population. It is frequently associated with hypertension. Although its exact cause and effect relationship with IHD has not yet been established, on the basis of the present state of medical knowledge doctors find it advisable to check uric acid levels of all cases of hypertension and to take corrective action, if the level is high.

Blood uric acid	Normal	up to 6 mg%
	Borderline	6-8 mg%
	Abnormal	above 8 mg %

(7) *Electrocardiogram (ECG)* is done to find out if there is any evidence of enlargement or hypertrophy of the heart, especially of the left ventricle, the chamber which mainly bears the brunt of the high blood pressure. The ECG may also

show evidence of a new or old heart attack or any disturbance of the rhythm of the heart. Ischaemia may be observed only in an ECG taken after exercise (stress test).

(8) *X-ray of the chest* gives the size of the heart and any signs of the failure of the functioning of the left ventricle such as congestion in the lungs.

Special Studies

These studies may have to be undertaken in the few selected patients in whom an underlying cause of hypertension is suspected. Since more than 90 per cent cases of hypertension are essential in nature, it is neither necessary nor cost-effective to submit every case to an expensive laboratory work up to rule out all the different causes of secondary hypertension. In general, it may be said that this may be necessary if hypertension is noticed before the age of twenty-five or after the age of sixty. Then the tests are tailored to individual requirement.

12

Goals and Principles of Treatment

The goal of treatment is simple—prevention of complications of hypertension, in order to ward off premature death and disability, increase lifespan and ensure a good quality of life. It has to be emphasised that the treatment is not directed towards symptoms of the disease, for the simple reason that these are few or none at all.

The complications which the treatment seeks to prevent have already been described in the previous pages. Briefly, they are:

- ischaemic heart disease—angina and heart attack;
- enlargement of the heart, mainly the left ventricle, and ultimately failure of its function (congestive heart failure);
- strokes, thrombotic and haemorrhagic, and paralysis;
- gangrene of the leg;
- malignant phase of hypertension; and
- damage to the eyes and kidneys.

You will appreciate that each one of these complications is serious and many are deadly, which can terminate life prematurely or cause lifelong incapacity resulting in dependence and a poor quality of life. It is, therefore, the duty of every hypertensive individual to keep his/her blood pressure under good control with the help of their physician.

What Treatment Can Do for You

There is a lot that treatment can achieve for you. For example:

- it prevents damage to target organs;
- to an extent, it can undo the damage already done;
- it can prevent the degeneration of arteries supplying blood to important organs;
- it can thus prevent such serious health problems as angina, heart attacks, strokes, kidney failure, etc; and
- it can prevent sudden spurts of blood pressure and thus ward off brain haemorrhage.

It thus helps to ensure longevity and good quality of life especially in later years.

Principles of Treatment

Treatment consists of:

(1) Physiological measures—readjustment in lifestyle, food, work, exercise, release of tension, etc. These measures, described in the next chapter, go a long way in lowering the blood pressure and correcting the associated metabolic abnormalities. They are enforced in all cases of hypertension, irrespective of its severity.

In mild and borderline cases, they alone may be sufficient to bring the desired result. If after 6 months of trial, desired reduction in blood pressure is not effected, drug therapy with antihypertensive drugs (Chapter 14) is added.

(2) Antihypertensive drugs—In all cases who have moderate or severe hypertension, physiological measures alone may not be sufficient to control the blood pressure to desirable level. Antihypertensive drugs are therefore started along with physiological measures but without waiting for their results.

It must be understood that blood pressure control is essential with physiological measures alone or with antihypertensive drugs added. Both lines of treatment have their own place and one cannot supplant the other.

13

Physiological Measures for Control of Hypertension

Our daily activities consist of working and resting, eating and drinking, sleeping, making love and so on.

It is important to know if what we are doing, on a lifetime basis, is right and correct as it ought to be. After all, there is nothing wrong in doing a bit of introspection to find out how our lifestyle affects our health and in particular blood pressure. Are we taking unnecessary and avoidable risks? Can we improve our lifestyle and make it more healthy for ourselves and our children? And this without losing the zest and pleasures of life. Life should be worth living, but at the same time we should not be unwittingly cutting it short for no cogent reason.

In this chapter, we shall try to find answers to these seemingly simple but important questions.

(I) WORK

I frequently hear statements like the following from my patients:

'Work has killed me.' 'Overwork was the cause of my blood pressure.' 'Too much work in the office caused my heart attack.'

It may be worth our while to examine if work really causes health problems and high blood pressure, and, if so, what to do about it.

The brain must think. This is the job for which it was created. If you do not give it good things to think about, it will think of mischief. Since it cannot remain idle, it will occupy itself with negative thoughts such as worry, anxiety, fear, jealously. These are unhealthy thoughts, not conducive to good health, happiness cr blood pressure. In fact, what cannot produce happiness cannot produce good blood pressure. It would, therefore, be wise to give the brain something constructive to think about.

Another point I wish to make is that whatever work is normal and natural for you is unlikely to cause adverse effects. The work that you like to do, the work for which you are trained, which is in accord with your nature, one which is not forced on you, which you do not have to do under threat, fear or tension, and one that is satisfying cannot cause ill-effects, for satisfying work does not produce stress. And what does not produce stress and strain does not contribute to hypertension.

What sort of work, then, produces hypertension? The work that produces tension and stress and is non-satisfying. It is the work that you do not like to do, the work which is not second nature to you, the one that is forced on you against your will or the one that is done under compulsion or fear, the work in which you are too time-bound, the work which you leave half done or the work which is postponed for no valid reason and which weighs on your mind, produces a rise in blood pressure.

While we have to strive not to get involved in a stressful work situation as far as possible, in today's competitive world it may not always be possible to be free from work that does not produce some stress or tension. However, you can do a great deal to reduce the tensions and keep your blood pressure under control. The following steps may be found useful:

- Do not keep your work pending.

- If you have to keep work pending, for reasons beyond your control, learn to be patient.
- Do not leave jobs half done.
- The job which needs a prolonged effort and cannot be done in a day, break it up into small daily units. That daily unit must not be left half done.
- You must aim at obtaining full satisfaction from your work. This presupposes that you have learnt your job well and do it to the best of your ability.
- Accept as much work as possible, but remember there are no more than 24 hours in a day; know your limitations.
- There is no better way to remove work tensions than to take at least an hour off daily, a day off in a week, and a fortnight off twice a year for rest, recreation and holiday.
- Forget your work routine and do not accept telephone calls during the period of your rest or holiday; you will come back refreshed and will work with double the vigour.
- Remember, satisfying work well done, interspersed with suitable periods of rest and recreation does not produce hypertension or heart disease. In fact, you should learn to enjoy your work.

(II) STRESS AND TENSION

The concept that modifying a patient's environment will help lower blood pressure is based on the theory that stressful environmental stimuli contribute to the elevation of blood pressure. Urban populations, which have to cope with considerably greater amounts of stress and strain, have higher levels of blood pressure than the rural folk. It is a common observation of doctors that a patient's blood pressure falls on admission to hospital without increase of medication; a busy executive on going on a holiday finds his blood pressure reduced. The reason for this is the removal from the stressful environment of the home or the work-place. While no controlled studies of the long-term effects of environmental change on blood pressure are yet available, the undoubted beneficial effect of such a change cannot be denied.

We live in the age of space, jets and computers. It is also the age of stress. Seven minutes past ten and ten minutes past ten make a difference to us. It was not so in our grandfather's time, when life was more leisurely. Our desires and ambitions are no longer as modest as theirs. The world has become highly competitive and we are all competitors, competing against one another.

How does this change affect our lives?

It certainly helps us to live better with more material comforts. But we all pay a price for it in the form of stress and high blood pressure.

What is Stress?

Stress is the result produced when the human body and mind are acted upon by forces that disrupt their equilibrium and produce strain. These adverse forces may be in the form of some injury; or psychological forces in the form of fear, anxiety or crisis. A certain amount of stress is probably necessary for our well-being and success in life. However, when stress occurs in quantities that our system cannot handle, it produces emotional disturbances and elevates blood pressure as well as causes certain pathological changes in the body resulting in such diseases as heart attacks, stomach ulcers, asthma, etc.

Man pays for his intelligence by way of prolonged stressful reactions, even when the cause of stress is no longer present. He sees danger which might never come. Our desires and ambitions do not let our mind and body rest and relax.

I know of an engineer, a brilliant inventor, who resigned his job, to start his own consultancy work. An extremely ambitious man, he was always working against time and overcoming obstacles. He suffered his first heart attack at fifty, but refused to change his hectic lifestyle and died of another heart attack at fifty-three.

He literally drove himself to death.

Contrast the engineer with another individual, an acquaintance of mine, whom I met twenty-five years ago, after a long gap. On a casual inquiry about his posting, I was surprised to learn that he had retired the previous month, meaning thereby that he had completed fifty-eight years of age. As a physician, I am used to assessing the age of my patients, and I had, in my mind, never placed him beyond the late forties. He looked at least ten years younger than his age, and was in excellent health. I was curious to know the reason behind his lasting youth. He told me that during his service career of more than thirty years he had always been lucky to get good bosses as well as good subordinates to work with, and never had problems with either. In fact, his own mental make-up and attitude to life were such that he never got himself into conflicts. He kept himself relaxed, worked reasonably hard and remained in good health, including his blood pressure. He is still alive, now in his eighties, and going strong.

These are two contrasting personalities, the former who was overly anxious, ambitious and working against time, driving himself towards health problems and an early death; and the other, relaxed and composed, never involving himself in conflicts and problems—a personality trait which has ensured good health and prolonged his life.

How to Cope with Stress

If you are hypertensive, the first thing you should do is to find out the areas of conflict, if any, and resolve them as far and as much as you can. Secondly, your ambitions have to be realistic. If you are well into middle age, you may have already realised them by now. But if this is not the case, there is no use fretting over it and continuing to make half-hearted efforts. It is much saner to accept reality. In the later years of your life, you have to live according to your age, not only physically but also mentally and emotionally. Ambitions in the later part of your life need to be consistent with your physical, mental and psychological capacity.

I am not suggesting a life of inactivity. Far from it, I am suggesting an active life till the end, one which is within your capacity, with reasonable periods of rest, recreation and holiday. I am suggesting that you keep a relaxed attitude of mind. What is important is not to work against time, not to be in a hurry, not to be too time-bound, not to look at the watch too often; in fact to go in for a little more leisurely and relaxed pace of work and activity with calm and composure, without losing your temper. In other words, I am asking you not to be at loggerheads with yourself (and others!) but to be your own friend. Keeping a calm and relaxed attitude of mind, free from confrontation and conflict, is not going to reduce the quality or output of your work. On the other hand, it will improve your work, and, most importantly, it will keep your blood pressure down. To this end hobbies, music and meditation may also help.

Relaxation by the Indian technique of meditation is becoming increasingly popular, not only in our own country, but also in the West. It is practised in many different forms. The principle is to use a mental device, which may be a *mantra,* a single word or a visual symbol, to relax the mind. By concentrating on this, to the exclusion of everything else, the body will start relaxing. In effect, it means giving the mind something fairly unexciting to think about, so as to blot out distracting thoughts. When such a thought enters the mind, it is replaced by the symbol or *mantra*. The technique is best learnt in a meditation centre. Many such centres are now functioning in almost all big towns in India and abroad.

(III) REST AND HOLIDAY

Rest

We have a lesson to learn from opium-eaters. It has been known for a long time that they have a long span of life. What is it that prolongs the life of an opium-eater in spite of the many unhealthy effects on the body and mind is an intriguing question. It is well known that opium-eaters are a lazy lot. They take life as it comes and are not bothered about trivialities. They do not exert much and never overexert. It is probably in this last fact that we have the answer to our query. You have already learnt that the arteries supplying blood to various organs, including the heart and brain, degenerate with age, and this process is hastened by hypertension. They cannot stand the strain of a sudden shooting up of the blood pressure and pulse and other body changes that occur on account of frayed tempers and outbursts of physical and emotional energy. In taking life lightly, the opium-eaters never overtax their capacity. They never enter, so to say, the danger zone of activity, be it physical, mental or emotional.

This is not to suggest that you should become an opium-eater to be able to live a long life. Far from that; such a life would not be worth living. But the lesson to learn is that as a hypertensive you should not be overtaxing and overshooting your physical and emotional capacity, especially as you grow in years. Remain well below the danger zone. Keep your cool, and work and exert within your capacity. Have adequate periods of rest. And when you feel tired or have adverse symptoms, give yourself extra rest. Never force yourself to go on exerting when your inner self says, 'It is too much'. Nobody except you will ever know when the exertion has become too much, just as only the wearer knows where the shoe pinches. Hear and pay heed to your inner voice. Don't ignore it. This is the opium-eater's message to you.

Leisure

Leisure is not laziness. It is spare time free from work and business. In a way it is earned by work. If your work is sedentary and tension-ridden, leisure is necessary to allow your brain to rest and relax as well as for your blood pressure to settle down. It is not a waste of time because it is necessary to streamline your thoughts. It may be fruitfully utilised in whatever interests you—reading, music, hobbies, friendly discussions or television viewing. It is time well spent.

Holiday

In today's competitive world there is nothing better than a holiday to release the tension built up during months of work in a stressful environment and thus favourably influence your blood pressure. The essential feature of a holiday is a change of environment. Just as sleep is essential after the day's work, a holiday is a requisite after some months of gruelling work. At a holiday you are at peace with yourself, away from your usual surroundings of the home and workplace. When you come back, your mind looks at things with a different perspective. Solutions to problems, which had eluded you earlier, spring to mind effortlessly. You feel light and bouyant and the work which had become a drudgery becomes interesting again. Both the quality of work and productivity improve. An all-round improvement in mutual relationships with people around you is noticed. All these factors are responsible for bringing down your elevated blood pressure in addition to an improvement in general health. All this because the body and mind have been given time to recover from the stresses and strains of city life. It may be pointed out that even if you live in a congenial environment and a comfortable home, a change of environment will still be found to be invigorating.

(IV) OBESITY

A clear link between hypertension and obesity, two of the major problems afflicting affluent classes in India, has been established. Obese persons are five times as likely to develop hypertension as the non-obese. Overweight hypertensives also suffer an increased incidence of complications of hypertension. Further, obese persons are more likely to develop diabetes, (another risk factor for the heart), degenerative joint pains and ligamentous aches.

Weight reduction is effective in reducing blood pressure and its complications. Weight control is, therefore, an important component of blood pressure management. But it needs to be emphasised that while it is beneficial to lose weight to ideal levels, it is not right to go down and then up the scale sometimes losing and then gaining weight. That is worse than not reducing at all. Therefore, after reducing, stay reduced.

Diagnosis

The diagnosis of obesity is usually a simple matter, even a glance may be sufficient. However, it is better evaluated by comparing the height and weight of the person with a standard chart (Appendix III).

A person who weighs more than the maximum permissible weight for his height is called overweight. And if he is 10 per cent (or 8 kg) or more overweight, he is termed obese.

How Obesity Produces Adverse Effects

An obese person carries an extra burden of inert fat. It is like carrying a bag of that much extra weight during the waking hours. Apart from the extra load placed on the weight-bearing joints and ligaments, it puts an extra burden on the heart and lungs, causing a person to get breathless. This makes him sluggish, causing a further reduction of physical activity, leading to more obesity. This becomes a vicious circle.

The unburnt fats raise the cholesterol level of blood, contributing to the development of fatty deposits (atheroma) in the major arteries of the heart and brain and are the cause of heart attacks and strokes (Chapter 9).

Can you Reduce the Risks by Shedding the Extra Weight?

The answer is best exemplified by this case. About ten years ago a prosperous factory owner in his late forties came to consult me about his heart condition. He was suffering from angina and shortness of breath condition. He was suffering from angina and shortness of breath on walking. He had already suffered one minor heart attack. He was very obese, more than 30 kg overweight. A vegetarian, he was very fond of sweets, parathas and other fried food, but had neither found the time nor the inclination for any physical work or exercise. With a fleet of cars at his disposal he had hardly felt the need to walk either for business or pleasure. We discussed the matter and he agreed to modify his diet and perform regular exercise. In about a year and a half, he shed all the extra weight, and in the process shed his angina too. Breathlessness on exertion also disappeared. He is now nearing sixty, has no serious health problem, and is hale and hearty.

Why do People Become Obese?

Your body weight depends upon how much you eat and how much you burn off the calories by physical work and exercise. If you eat less and work more, you lose weight. Conversely, if you eat more and work less, you gain weight. The extra calories are converted by the body into fat and stored. Over the years you accumulate more and more fat and become obese.

Is it Enough to Reduce Intake of Fats?

Consuming fats—ghee, butter, vegetable oils—is of course fattening. But this is not the whole story. Consumption of sweets, sugar, rice, chapattis, potatoes and other carbohydrates also contributes to weight gain because our diet contains large amounts of these foodstuffs. Our body converts the unutilised or unspent calories from carbohydrates into fats. The worst offender in our diet is fried food like parathas and purees which contain both carbohydrates and fat, and which stimulate the appetite, leading to overeating.

Are There Any Drugs to Reduce Weight?

There are no useful or safe drugs for reducing weight. The only way to shed weight is to eat less and work more. By work I mean physical work and exercise (see section V of this chapter).

Weight Reducing Diet

The diet should contain enough proteins, which are body building substances, but carbohydrates and fats should be cut down. The diet should be such that it contains enough vitamins and minerals.

All fried food should be abstained from. Pulses and milk along with some poultry and fish for non-vegetarians will supply all the necessary proteins. Take fresh vegetables and fruits in plenty; they are good sources of vitamins and minerals. Take plenty of salads, which are stomach fillers and also supply plenty of fibre along with vitamins. Take water or diluted buttermilk (*lassi*) before you begin eating, so that the stomach becomes partly full. You will eat less this way. Take only small helpings of rice or chapatti, the main source of carbohydrates in our food.

On this diet you will not only reduce your weight but also your blood pressure.

How Much Weight Reduction per Month should be Aimed at?

If you aim to lose 1 to 1½ kg per month, you will encounter no difficulty. But if you are very obese, you should aim at losing about 2 kg per month. This way you will shed 10-15 kg in a year.

Crash Diets

Crash diets are not easy to practise and are likely to cause deficiencies of vitamins and minerals. They may lead to a great deal of weakness, which may interfere with your work. They cannot be maintained for long, so there is a greater likelihood of obesity coming back. As said earlier, it is not right to go down and up the scale.

It is much better, easier and healthier to aim at reasonable monthly targets. The great advantage in doing so is that by the time you have shed the extra weight you will become accustomed to the reduced diet. With slight adjustments, such a diet can (and should) be maintained indefinitely so that obesity does not return.

Role of Fasting

Fasting on specific days of the week may be helpful, provided you do not overeat on the next day. Long periods of fasting at a stretch are inadvisable.

Vitamin Supplements During Dieting

If crash diets are not practised and if the diet is well balanced, as indicated above, vitamin supplements may not be necessary. But in practice it is not always possible to ensure an adequate intake of vitamins and trace elements, so necessary for good health. It may, therefore, be worthwhile to take a daily supplement of vitamins and minerals, such as Becadexamine, Supradyn, Multibionta. One tablet/capsule daily is more than enough.

The important point to remember in the control of obesity is the old adage, "Slow and steady wins the race."

Prevention of Obesity

It has to be admitted that treatment of obesity is slow and time-consuming. The difficulty of treating obesity in adults and the observation that adult obesity is related to childhood ponderosity clearly suggest that its prevention at an early age might be a better option than attempting a cure in later life.

We have in our bodies depots of adipose (fatty) tissue under the skin and abdomen. The amount of fat that we can collect depends upon the number and size of fat cells in the body. Studies have identified two critical periods for proliferation of the adipose tissue. First and more important is before the age of two, and the second is during the adolescent growth spurt. It is now believed that breast-feeding of babies, in preference to formula or cow's milk, prevents proliferation of adipose tissue and protects against later obesity and diabetes. If prudent dietary practices are then pursued at home during childhood and adolescence, adult obesity can be prevented. For prevention of obesity and the future health of your children:

(a) Breast-feed them;
(b) enforce prudent dietary practices during their childhood and adolescence, which should be continued indefinitely. (See section X of this chapter).

(V) EXERCISE AND PHYSICAL ACTIVITY

The lifestyle of the hypertensive is invariably marked by sedentary work and little exercise. In what way exercise helps mitigate the adverse effects of such a lifestyle and those of hypertension shall be examined in this section. We shall also discuss what type and how much of exercise is right for you.

What is Exercise?

Exercise does not only mean tennis and football or walking and jogging. Any physical activity is exercise. If you are a house-wife doing all the household work yourself, including cleaning floors, washing clothes, preparing meals, etc., it may give you enough exercise. Similarly, if you walk to your office and back, covering a few kilometres or, if as a physician you have to take long rounds of the hospital wards, it is an exercise.

What is Achieved by Exercise?

Exercise helps lower blood pressure. It helps prevent adverse effects of other factors which may be associated with hypertension. It raises the beneficial HDL-cholesterol; it helps burn sugar and fats, thus, preventing obesity, and corrects sugar metabolism. In this manner it helps prevent complications of hypertension like heart attacks.

What and How Much Exercise?

All physical activity has to be undertaken keeping in view your age and general physical health, particularly that of your heart. As a general rule, physical activity may be unrestricted below the age of about thirty-five years. After that age, it should be gradually toned down to become less and less strenuous as age advances. If indulging in games, hypertensives would do well to play for the sake of fun and exercise only and not for that of competition. All competitive games should be discontinued. This is particularly important if heart problems make their appearance. After the age of about sixty, the only correct type of exercise is walking at a comfortable pace.

Precautions

Whatever the physical activity, tennis, badminton, walking or jogging or household chores, it is important to remember that while exercise is good for hypertensives, excessive or unaccustomed exercise can be harmful. The following precautions are suggested:

- Do not take unaccustomed exercise, accustom yourself first by starting at a lower level of exercise and gradually increase the intensity and duration.
- At any level of exercise you should not become unduly breathless or feel unduly tired or feel tired for an unduly prolonged period.
- The correct intensity and duration of exercise is one that gives you a pleasant feeling of tiredness which disappears after resting for a while.
- If the exercise produces any pain in the chest, even of a short duration, or any other untoward symptom, consult your doctor before proceeding with the exercise; he may like to investigate your heart.
- Do not take exercise at a time when your blood pressure is uncontrolled and excessively elevated, but rest.

- If you have not been taking any exercise earlier and wish to start an exercise programme, first discuss with your doctor.

(VI) SEXUAL ACTIVITY

Is sexual activity safe for hypertensives, and if so, to what extent? This is an important question as it concerns the intimate life of every patient. It, therefore, needs a clear-cut answer.

Sexual Activity in Uncomplicated Hypertension

Sexual activity is like any other normal human activity. It has the advantage of releasing tension and keeping the mind in balance. To this extent, it is useful in lowering blood pressure. However, during sexual intercourse there is a sudden and abrupt rise of heart (pulse) rate and blood pressure, though for a brief period. If the blood pressure is uncontrolled and very high before the act, it can go up to dangerous levels and can cause complications like a heart attack or stroke. With a properly controlled blood pressure the sexual activity should do no harm; in fact is should be useful.

Sexual Activity when Complications are Present

If complications of hypertension, e.g., angina or heart attack, have occurred, such cases will have to be individually assessed by the physician. In general terms the following line of action may be desirable : In case there is angina but there has been no damage to the heart by way of a heart attack and angina is well controlled with medication, moderate sexual activity which does not precipitate chest pain or undue breathlessnes may be indulged in. Precautions mentioned below may be useful.

Even in case heart attack has already occurred, sexual activity can be resumed sooner or later by almost 80-90 per cent of patients. These patients will have to be carefully assessed for their fitness by the physician. When they have achieved good exercise tolerance and no adverse symptoms or disturbances of heart rhythm or adverse changes in ECG are produced by exercise, they would be considered fit to resume a normal sex life. This may take a few months after the heart attack. As a rough indication, the ability to go up a flight of stairs at a good speed without producing adverse symptoms of chest pain, palpitations or unduly prolonged breathlessness is good enough for resuming normal sexual intercourse.

Can the Sex Act Precipitate a Heart Attack?

Studies have shown that in the course of normal daily activities there are many occasions when the heart rate and blood pressure rise to as high or even higher levels than those attained during normal sexual intercourse, for instance, while driving a scooter in a crowded, traffic-infested market-place. In a hypertensive, the risk of precipitating a heart attack during normal sexual intercourse is, therefore, no greater than during the performance of normal daily activities. But what is important are the circumstances attendant on sexual intercourse.

What are those circumstances? Sexual activity in the confines of the home in the marital bed with a sympathetic wife as the partner is just another human function. Contrast this with clandestine sex in a hotel room with a strange partner to whom one's potency has to be proved. There may have been much smoking and drinking prior to the act. Further, the anxiety and fear of being found out coupled with feelings of guilt could make matters worse. All these factors produce a much greater strain and increase many times the chances of precipitating a heart attack or even sudden death.

Precautions

- Avoid intercourse soon after meals, wait for at least four hours after a meal, this is the time required for the digestive processes to take effect, when much of the blood is diverted to the abdomen leaving less for the use of the heart.

- If certain positions are found too strenuous or exhausting or tend to produce adverse symptoms, change the position to a less strenuous one.
- Alternatively, let your spouse play the more active role.
- Betablocking drugs, like Inderal, are used to treat hypertension. They also act as cardio-protective agents by preventing the heart rate and blood pressure from rising too high. A suitable dose an hour or so before the act may prevent the blood pressure and heart rate from shooting up and thus prevent the possibility of a heart attack or brain haemorrhage. This measure is especially important if ischaemic heart disease coexists or if the hypertension is severe. Your doctor will be able to advise you regarding the correct dose for you after ascertaining that no contraindication to its use exists in your case.
- Above all, avoid clandestine sex, which can be most dangerous.

(VII) NON-ALCOHOLIC BEVERAGES

Among the non-alcoholic beverages, tea and coffee are popular the world over to remove fatigue and give gentle stimulation and warmth. Cola drinks are also popular in warmer climates for the same purpose. Chocolate drinks, like Bournvita and Ovaltine in milk are commonly consumed as a nightcap.

Effects on the Body

The common denominator of all these drinks is caffein and other xanthines, which are responsible for the effects we seek. Caffein stimulates the brain, body and the heart. It removes fatigue and sleep, and improves performance. It causes a transient rise of blood pressure and makes the heart work faster. It increases the secretion of urine.

Excessive and prolonged consumption of xanthines causes marked increase in the heart rate and irregularity of heart action (extrasystoles). These effects result in palpitations. The blood pressure may by elevated persistently, along with a sense of anxiety, restlessness, headache and loss of sleep. Coffee, when taken in excessive quantities, has particularly undesirable effects. It increases blood cholesterol. Epidemiological studies suggest increased risk of angina and heart attacks, and a possible link with cancer of the pancreas.

Should Hypertensives Drink Caffeinated Beverages?

These beverages give a great deal of satisfaction to a large number of people. Except for coffee, if consumed in excess, there is no evidence of harmful effects and all the evidence of favourable effects when taken in moderation. Consumed in moderate quantities, the effect on blood pressure is only transient. There is, therefore, no objection to hypertensive patients drinking moderate quantities of these beverages, especially tea. Heavy coffee drinking should be avoided by them in view of the possible adverse effects on the heart.

What is a Heavy Consumption?

Consumption of more than 300 mg of caffein by normal young people and 200 mg by the hypertensive or the elderly is termed excessive. Each cup of coffee contains about 80 mg, a cup of tea about 30 mg and a bottle of a cola drink about 30 mg of caffein. So you can calculate what is excessive for you.

What is a Safe and Moderate Consumption?

If you take 3 or 4 cups of tea and a cup of coffee or a cola drink in a day, it should be both safe and satisfying. However, the elderly may better avoid these drinks in the evenings lest they interfere with their sleep. A chocolate drink (Bournvita, Ovaltine, etc.) as a nightcap is most unsuitable as it may have just the opposite effect in many persons and disturb their sleep. Restful sleep is necessary for hypertensives and helps in the proper control of their blood pressure. Therefore, anything interfering with sleep must be avoided.

(VIII) ALCOHOLIC DRINKS

In the struggle for happiness and warding off misery, man has invented many intoxicating substances, the foremost among them being alcohol. It ranks so high with men and societies the world over that they have given it an established place in their lifestyle. The value of alcohol in making social intercourse easy and pleasant cannot be denied, but the feeling of immediate pleasure and independence of the outer world that it provides are the very qualities which constitute the menace and the scourge that it is for mankind.

Adverse Effects on Blood Pressure

Regular consumption of alcohol in moderate to large quantities has far-reaching adverse effects on almost all the systems of the body, and is associated with increased incidence of hypertension, particularly systolic. While in large quantities alcohol has a direct constricting effect on the blood vessels, causing the blood pressure to rise, and acute elevation of blood pressure is known to occur after a bout of alcohol, the exact cause of the association of sustained hypertension and alcoholism remains unknown. The worst part is that the blood pressure may also rise on withdrawal of alcohol.

Alcohol is also known to cause serious reactions when combined with certain drugs—disulfiram (Antabuse); Flagyl, Tinidazole (drugs used for dysentery), and oral antidiabetic drugs. The reaction consists of an acute fall of blood pressure, difficulty in breathing, chest pain, nausea and vomiting. This reaction with Antabuse has been used to induce alcohol withdrawal but can be dangerous.

Beneficial Effects

Alcohol has some beneficial effects too, but only if consumed in small quantities, equivalent to about 20 gm of absolute alcohol. In this quantity it has been seen to alleviate anxiety and nervous tension and dilate peripheral blood vessels thus helping in reducing blood pressure. Further, in small quantities it increases the HDL-cholesterol in the blood, which is beneficial for the heart and protects it from heart attacks. Translated into alcoholic beverages, 20 gm of alcohol is equivalent to about 50 ml of spirits like whisky and brandy, 150 ml of wines and about 500 ml of beer. If anyone who drinks, restricts himself to this amount daily, with two alcohol free days in a week to allow regenerative processes to take effect, he will in all probability be gaining all the benefits that alcohol is capable of giving without its deleterious effects.

Should Teetotaller Hypertensives be Given the Benefit of Alcohol?

This is a frequently asked question, and the answer is a big 'No'. No doctor would advise a teetotaller to start drinking (even if he himself drinks!). There are sound reasons for this assertion. First, the few beneficial effects far outweigh the long list of ill-effects. Second, all the beneficial effects can be obtained by a much safer and cheaper way, e.g., regular exercise. Third, even in small quantities alcohol contributes to serious road accidents; no amount is safe for driving. Fourth, consumption of alcohol even in small quantities may not be entirely safe for the liver, particularly if it has sustained some previous injury. Lastly, the most serious problem with alcohol is that nobody can predict with any degree of certainty which person on starting to drink will become an alcoholic. No, the teetotallers, hypertensive or not, are best off without it.

Summing Up

- Small quantities of alcohol are helpful in lowering blood pressure and protect the heart.
- Quantities greater than 50 ml of whisky or brandy, 150 ml of wines or 500 ml of beer per day with two alcohol-free days in a week should not be consumed.

- Regular consumption of larger amounts of alcohol adversely affects all body systems and is associated with increased incidence of hypertension.
- Alcohol combined with certain drugs can cause serious reaction such as a severe fall in blood pressure, chest pain and vomiting. The reactions can be dangerous.
- All the benefits of alcohol far outweigh its deleterious effects and these benefits can be obtained by safer and cheaper means, e.g., exercise.
- Teetotallers are best off without alcohol.

(IX) SMOKING

Ever since Columbus brought tobacco from the New World of America five centuries ago, it rapidly spread all over Europe and the rest of the world. Man's search for contentment and relief from boredom, and the rapid and strong habit-forming nature of its alkaloid, nicotine, have made smoking the menace that it is to mankind. In spite of the ever-increasing taxation and prices of cigarettes and the statutory warnings on every pack, cigarette smoking continues to be a popular pastime in all societies the world over.

Does Smoking Adversely Affect Hypertension?

It is a fact that the blood pressure rises for a short while after a cigarette. Though there is no evidence available to say that it contributes to the production of sustained elevation of blood pressure, it is also a fact that hypertensives who smoke are more liable to develop malignant phase of hypertension (chapter 10, vi) which takes them rapidly on a downhill course.

Hypertension itself is a serious risk factor for the heart, and so is nicotine. Nicotine increases fatty acids and cholesterol in the blood, and reduces the beneficial HDL-cholesterol. These alterations facilitate the formation of fatty deposits (atheroma) in the major arteries of the heart, brain, legs, etc., thus facilitating and increasing the incidence of angina, heart attacks, strokes, and gangrene of the leg. Further, nicotine increases the heart (pulse) rate and causes irregular action of the heart by producing extra beats (extrasystoles). The carbon monoxide in the smoke combines with the haemoglobin in the blood to form inert carboxy-haemoglobin which cannot carry oxygen. The body, heart and brain, in particular, are thus deprived of oxygen. This worsens angina.

Recent research has found that smoking has a synergistic effect with hypertension, as well as a direct effect in the causation of strokes, i.e,. cerebral infraction and subarachnoid haemorrhage. The relative risk of strokes among heavy smokers who are hypertensive is five times that of smokers who have a normal blood pressure, and 20 times of those who are non-smokers and have normal blood pressure. The risk increases as the number of cigarettes smoked rise. Cessation of smoking reduces the risk. It becomes substantially less after two years and reaches the level of non-smokers after five years. Heavy smokers with hypertension stand to benefit most from stopping smoking and controlling their blood pressure.

Apart from the above adverse effects on the cardiovascular system, smoking is linked to many other serious disease conditions, such as:

—cancers of the lung and mouth
—chronic bronchitis and emphysema
—respiratory insufficiency
—congestive heart failure.

Therefore, every hypertensive is well advised to abstain from smoking regardless of the level of his blood pressure. Contrary to the usual belief, it is not difficult to stop smoking. Only one in seven persons, usually women, find any real difficulty. All said and done, the easiest and the best thing to do is not to start smoking in the first place.

(X) FOOD FOR THE HYPERTENSIVE

Are there any foods which are particularly harmful or specifi-cally beneficial to the hypertensive, is an important question, on the answer of which depends the food policy that you have to adopt.

At the outset, I must allay the fear that there is no food in common use, consuming which can cause a sudden elevation or precipitate a fall of blood pressure. There is no such effect like a high sugar or carbohydrate diet producing an immediate rise of blood sugar in a diabetic patient. What we are looking for are the long-term effects of food on the blood pressure and its complications.

Our food policy should be such as to take care of two factors, namely, the level of blood pressure, and the prevention/correction of metabolic abnormalities of salt, cholesterol, obesity and glucose, any of which may be associated with hypertension and act as risk factors for the heart and other organs.

Role of Salt

It has long been known that a high consumption of salt (sodium chloride) produces a rise of blood pressure and, conversely, low consumption produces a fall (Chapter 7). The effect does not only depend upon the common salt that we add to our food but also upon the sodium chloride that is naturally present in foodstuffs. Half a century ago, when we had no medicines to lower the blood pressure the only way doctors tried to control the blood pressure of their patients was by advising a salt-free rice diet (rice contains the lowest salt content of its own). Now that effective medicines are available, we no longer have to submit our patients to the rigors of a salt-free diet. But the lesson of the story is that the patient should take a low-salt diet and avoid highly salted food. The total salt content of the food should not exceed about 6 gm per day, including the natural salt content of the food. Normal food without added salt contains about half this amount. So you can add about 3 gm (½ to ⅔ teaspoonful) per day. I would suggest that your wife cooks your food without adding salt. Make a small paper packet of about half a teaspoon of common salt as your day's ration. Use it in any manner you like. If you are a rice-eater, you can afford to increase this ration to about one teaspoon.

Small as it is, there are simple ways to be happy with this ration :

- The amount of salt you need is directly proportional to the amount of chillies and spices in the food. Stop putting chillies in the food and the consumption of salt will automatically reduce.
- Leave the gravy in the dish uneaten.
- Make dishes without gravy as far as possible. Sprinkle a few crystals of salt on top, but don't mix. When eating, the crystals will come in direct contact with your taste buds. The latter will be deceived into believing that the food has plenty of salt.
- Indian pickles, achars and chutneys contain very large amounts of salt; avoid them.

The taste buds, which were accustomed to a high-salt diet, gradually regain their sensitivity to salt in a few weeks' time. You will then feel satisfied with your ration.

Role of Potassium, Magnesium and Calcium

It is also now known that low potassium content in the food elevates the blood pressure. In effect, it is the balance between sodium and potassium which appears to be important. A diet rich in sodium and poor in potassium tends to elevate the blood pressure, while a low-salt high-potassium diet tends to lower it. Potassium is contained in most of the vegetables and fruits. Bananas and citrus fruits (orange, malta, kinu, mossammi) are particularly rich in it.

Calcium and magnesium are also considered important to keep the blood pressure under control. These too are found in vegetables, fruits and milk. Appendix II gives you the common sources of these minerals.

If you eat a lot of vegatables and fruits, milk and yoghurt, along with low consumption of common salt, you will have the correct balance of sodium and potassium along with adequate quantities of magnesium and calcium, which will help your blood pressure to stay at lower levels. In any case, it will appreciably reduce the need and dose of antihypertensive drugs. Don't forget to remove the layer of cream (malai) from milk and yoghurt.

Role of Fibre

A recent study of more than 30,000 health care professionals, 40 to 75 years of age, conducted by the Harvard School of Public Health, has confirmed the role diet plays in controlling the blood pressure. It supports the concept that eating a lot of fruits and vegetables helps prevent hypertension. The study ascribes the beneficial effects to the fibre contained in vegetarian foods. Incidentally, such a diet is helpful for diabetics too.

Foods Affecting Risk Factors Associated with Hypertension

High blood cholesterol and obesity, commonly associated with hypertension, are risk factors for the heart. Heavy consumption of fats, particularly animal fats like eggs, butter and ghee, is responsible. Eggs have the highest cholesterol content in the yolk, the yellow part. Hypertensive patients would do well to cut down the consumption of eggs and animal fats, and use vegetable oils instead as the cooking medium. It needs to be highlighted that so far as obesity is concerned, both animal as well as vegetable fats are equally likely to cause it. The consumption of vegetable fats should not, therefore, be excessive. For warding off obesity, it is also important to keep the consumption of sugar, sweets and carbohydrates to less than moderate levels, and to avoid fried foods like parathas altogether. These measures will also help prevent disorders of sugar metabolism and help control diabetes, if present.

Conclusion

From the above discussion it would be obvious that for a patient of hypertension or a member of a hypertensive family, the correct diet is a low-salt vegetarian diet with plenty of fresh vegetables and fruits; rice is the preferred staple cereal. Consumption of animal fats and eggs, should be cut down; vegetable oil, which does not solidify in the North Indian winter, should be used as the preferred cooking medium but in modest quantities. Milk and yoghurt from which the creamy layer has been removed should be taken freely.

It may be added in the end that while the major portion of the food should consist of vegetables, fruits and cereals, non-vegetarian items of food need not be completely removed from the diet. Fish is positively beneficial, chicken is acceptable, while red meat (lamb, pork, beef) needs to be restricted, but organ meat (brain, liver, etc.) should be avoided altogether because of its high cholesterol content. With this exception, non-vegetarian foods cannot be called harmful for the hypertensive. It is the exclusion of fruits and vegetables from the diet which is harmful.

In a Nutshell

A hypertensive's diet should comprise the following:

- Plenty of fresh vegetables and fruits,
- cereals (rice is the preferred cereal),
- milk from which cream has been skimmed off, and
- nuts and seeds.

For the non-vegetarian, plenty of the above plus the following:

- Fish and chicken in moderation,
- occasionally red meat (mutton, pork, beef), and
- eggs, restricted to 5 per week.

A hypertensive should avoid:

- Tinned vegetables as they contain much salt
- organ meat (liver, brain, etc.).

All food should be prepared without salt; the daily ration of salt (½-1 teaspoon) can be sprinkled over.

14

Drugs Used in the Treatment of Hypertension

I will now briefly describe the drugs used in the treatment of hypertension as well as the care and precautions necessary in their use. I may, however, emphasise the fact that the treatment responsibility, the choice of the drugs and their dosage are entirely at the discretion of the physician. This chapter is written merely for the information of the reader to enable him to give full cooperation to his physician.

In the first half of this century, till about 1950, we had no drugs which could lower elevated blood pressure. The only treatment known to help hypertensive patients was a salt-free rice diet. I was a young doctor in those days. A doctor colleague, who was hypertensive, could do nothing to reduce his blood pressure and he would not take the insipid salt-free rice diet. One day his blood pressure shot up to 240/140. He became unconscious and showed signs of paralysis. Luckily, he recovered in a short time; it was not thrombosis but encephalopathy due to the sudden and precipitate rise of blood pressure. He was strongly advised to take a salt-free rice diet—the only thing we could advise in those days. His blood pressure came down to safer levels but to nowhere near normal. I can't forget how miserable he used to feel taking such a tasteless insipid diet day in and day out, but what could we do? We had nothing better to offer him.

The first drug for reduction of blood pressure, Reserpine (Serpasil), was introduced in 1950, you will he happy to know by an Indian physician, Rustom Jal Vakil. It was prepared from an Indian herb, *Rauwolfia serpentina.* This herb had been used in India for centuries to treat mental illness and anxiety. It reduces blood pressure and acts as a tranquiliser. Reserpine is still used occasionally, usually in combination with other drugs. It sometimes causes depression and has to be withdrawn.

Over the years better and more effective drugs have been introduced. Now, a variety of useful drugs are available to the physician for use in his hypertensive patients.

Oral Diuretics and Beta-blocking Drugs

The most extensively used drugs have been oral diuretics and beta-blockers. They were among the first to arrive on the scene, easy-to-use, reasonably safe for long-term use and relatively inexpensive.

Diuretics are used not for their urine secreting effect, but their effect of throwing out salt (sodium chloride) through the urine. So, the salt depleting effect is still used today to lower the blood pressure. Though we no longer submit our patients to the rigors of the insipid salt-free rice diet, we still insist on a low-salt diet.

The diuretics throw out potassium in addition to salt (sodium), so that potassium supplements have to be given, either in the form of a syrup or a capsule or citrus fruits. Potassium depletion can be harmful, even dangerous, especially for the heart if a heart attack occurs. However, certain diuretics have been introduced which conserve potassium, so that a mixture of potassium-losing and potassium-conserving diuretics (Dytide, Biduret) are frequently prescribed by doctors.

The beta-blockers—Propranolol (Inderal), Atenolol (Betanol, Betacard), Acebutolol (Sectral), Lebetalol (Normadate), etc.— were the next to arrive. They reduce the heart (pulse) rate and reduce the strength of contraction of the heartbeat. They thus reduce the blood pressure and at the same time protect the heart against inordinate rise of pulse rate and strain as, for example, during sexual intercourse. They are also used to treat angina and for cardioprotection after a heart attack.

Individually, diuretics and beta-blockers are not powerful hypotensive agents, but given together they are reasonably effective against mild or moderate hypertension. Unfortunately, recent research has pointed out certain adverse effects. Many of the diuretics and beta-blockers adversely affect the lipid profile of patients on long-term use. They either raise the blood cholesterol, particularly LDL-cholesterol, or lower the beneficial HDL-cholesterol. These changes tend to increase the patient's chances of getting complications of hypertension like a heart attack or a stroke. Hence, the initial enthusiasm for these drugs has now cooled down. They are no longer considered as first-line drugs against hypertension as they used to be. However, they are still considered useful for short-term use or in lower doses as an adjunct to other drugs.

Hydrallazine (Neprisol) is a relatively older drug. It has the advantage of being inexpensive, not a small consideration for lifelong treatment. It is still in use, usually in combination with a beta-blocker or diuretic and rescrpine in small doses.

Methyl-dopa (Aldomet, Emdopa), also an older drug, is still in use, especially in complications of hypertension during pregnancy. Its sleep-inducing effect sometimes interferes with the patient's work and can be dangerous while driving, but is not a disadvantage during pregnancy or at night.

Clonidine (Catapres, Hyperdine) is a drug of the seventies. It also produces somnolence. It has one great drawback: suddenly stopping it or missing a dose or two can cause rebound hypertension, and the level of blood pressure may go skyrocketting with all the attendant dangers like cerebral haemorrhage.

Calcium channel blockers, especially Nifedipine (Calbloc, Calcigard, Nifedine) and its analogues, Felodipine (Renedil) and Amlodipine (Amlogard, Tamlod) are currently the most favoured class of drugs used against hypertension. Nifedipine is usually prescribed in sustained release long-acting form, and is usually combined with a small amount of a beta-blocker, Atenolol. Since both these drugs are anti-anginal, and cardioprotective, they are useful if angina coexists.

The last to arrive on the therapeutic scene are ACE-inhibitors—Captopril (Aceten), Enalepril (Envas, En-Ace), Lisinopril (Lisoril), etc. They are useful for patients who are not adequately responding to calcium channel blockers.

Precautions (See chapter 20).

The treatment of every patient has to be individualised, both regarding the choice of drugs as well as the dosage. This is the job of the physician. You, as a patient, cannot and should not fix or change the dose nor should you change the prescribed drug on your own. After all, these are potent drugs and cannot be treated like popcorn.

It must be clearly understood that there is no treatment available yet which can radically cure essential hypertension. The treatment consists of lifelong control of the disease, repeat, lifelong. Taking treatment for a few days or months and then stopping it serves no purpose.

Physiological and drug treatments are complementary to each other. Even if your blood pressure is well controlled with drugs, adjustments in lifestyle are an equally important part of blood pressure management and may be the only treatment necessary if your blood pressure is controlled around 140/90.

Proper control of your blood pressure is imperative whether achieved by physiological measures alone or with the addition of drugs. For this purpose, observation by your doctor is essential. When you need to consult him is indicated in Chapter 20.

15

Potential Problems of Medication

The anti-hypertensive drugs started arriving on the scene only after 1950. The earlier drugs had troublesome side-effects. In spite of these effects, they had to be used because they were lesser evil than the disease. The newer drugs are comparatively free from these problems, and it is now possible to treat hypertensive patients with fair degree of ease and without interference in their work or love life. However, minor effect may sometimes occur, or it may sometimes be necessary to use older drugs for special effects or advantages in particular situations. You should therefore be aware of these unwanted actions so that you can take timely action or report to your doctor for suitable reduction of dose or modification of therapy. The following table will give you the necessary information:

Group	Common Examples	Common Trade Names	Common Side-effects	Action required
Diuretics	Chlorthalidone Hydrochlorthiazide	Hythaltone Esidrex	Weakness, muscle cramps, impotence, frequent urination, sun sensitivity	Orange juice; reduction of dose.
Beta-Blockers	Propranolol Atenolol Metoprolol	Inderal Betacard Tenolol Betaloc Metolar	Nightmares, insomnia weakness, dizziness, cold hand and feet, impotence, worsening of asthma	Reduction of dose or change of therapy.

contd.

ACE-Inhibitors	Captopril Enalepril Lisinopril	Aceten Envas Lisoril	Loss of taste, unaccounted cough, palpitations, headache, rashes	Dose reduction or change of drug.
Calcium-Channel-Blockers	Diltiazem Nifedipine Amlodipine	Dilzem Depin Amcard	Swelling of legs, dizziness, headaches, hot flushes, constipation, palpitations	Elastic bandage on legs; increase excercise and fibre in diet, small dose of beta-blocker.
Alpha-Blockers	Prazosin Terazosin	Prazopress Hytrin	First dose hypotension, faintness.	First dose not to exceed half; Avoid abrupt movements.
Vasodilators	Dihydralazine	Nepresol	Headaches, palpitations, rapid heart rate.	Reduction of dose; addition of Betablocker.
Centrally Acting Alpha-Blockers	Clonidine Methyldopa	Catapres Aldomet	Dry mouth, drowsiness, fatigue, constipation, Reactive hypertension with stoppage of clonidine.	Increase fluid intake; don't drive or work on machines when drowsy; reduction of dose; Never stop clonidine abruptly or miss a dose.
Peripherally Acting Adrenergic Antagonists	Reserpine	Serpasil	Depression, nightmares, stuffy nose, impotence.	Change of therapy.

16

Hypertension in the Elderly

Treatment of hypertension for those above the age of about sixty-five years needs special mention. By this age fatty deposits (atheromas) have developed at many places in the arterial tree. These deposits may not be large enough to produce obstruction to the flow of blood and may not, therefore, be causing any symptoms or problems. But when the blood pressure is lowered, obstruction in the blood flow may develop, especially in the arteries of the brain, resulting in ischaemia, i.e., lack of blood supply. The patient may fall down unconscious or develop adverse symptoms related to the nervous system.

In the elderly, therefore, doctors do not bring down the blood pressure abruptly, but gradually. Doses of antihypertensive drugs are suitably lowered so that the diastolic pressure does not fall much below 90 mm. In fact, 150/92 is the optimal blood pressure to be maintained in the elderly.

Systolic hypertension is common in the elderly. In them, special care has to be taken while lowering the blood pressure so as to avoid excessive fall of diastolic fall.

In elderly males, enlargement of the prostate gland is common. This causes some degree of obstruction to the flow of urine, leading to stasis of urine in the urinary bladder and infection.

The infection may be mild but chronic. Such chronic urinary tract infections tend to keep the blood pressure high, and their treatment and eradication may itself lower the blood pressure. The treatment usually consists of suitable and prolonged antibiotic therapy, but the recurrence of infection may indicate the necessity of surgical removal of the enlarged gland.

17

Hypertension in Pregnancy

Hypertension in a pregnant woman may be a matter of serious import and, therefore, it needs special mention. It may threaten the life of the mother as well as cause the birth of a small baby who may be suffocated or stillborn.

Hypertension can implicate pregnancy for three reasons; first, pregnancy may occur in a hypertensive woman; second, toxaemia of pregnancy (pre-eclampsia) may occur in a previously normotensive woman; third, pre-eclampsia may complicate pre-existing hypertension.

In the first case, when pregnancy occurs in an already hypertensive woman, all that is required is a readjustment of treatment because certain antihypertensive drugs may be unsuitable for use in pregnancy or unsafe for the unborn child, (e.g., ACE-inhibitors, beta-blockers) and the patient put on suitable drugs like methyl-dopa (Aldomet). Normally, with the proper control of blood pressure such patients go through pregnancy quite well. However, if pre-eclampsia supervenes on top of the pre-existing hypertension, it becomes a matter for concern.

In the second and third cases, hypertension (along with headache and swelling of ankles) occurs as a direct result of pregnancy, usually after the 20th week. This hypertension causes great anxiety because it may pose a danger to the life o«p-3Xf the mother as well as adversely affect the development of the foetus. Doctors control the hypertension, perform repeated urine examinations to see if any adverse changes (protein) appear therein, as the kidneys are the principal target organ to suffer, the others being the liver and blood. In pre-eclampsia, blood pressure readings even lower than usually considered to be dangerous can cause serious damage, including brain haemorrhage. Severe jaundice and coagulation of blood within the arteries are other serious manifestations of the disease process.

Doctors try to keep the blood pressure below 170/110, but in case the blood pressure cannot be kept under control or the urine shows evidence of kidney damage or serious symptoms threaten the life of the woman, the pregnancy may have to be terminated. Effort is made to keep the pregnancy going till the foetus is at least viable, though premature. But if this is not possible due to danger to the mother, the foetus may have to be sacrificed to save the mother. This is probably the strongest medical indication for the termination of pregnancy. As soon as pregnancy is terminated or delivery takes place, the blood pressure returns to normal and the danger to the mother recedes.

Apart from the control of blood pressure, low dose aspirin, just about 60 mg (1/6 tablet) per day, is the first medical treatment which has been shown to prevent or retard effectively the development of pre-eclampsia, though its safety to the unborn child and the pregnant mother is yet to be defined.

18

Hypertensive Families

It is a well known fact that in certain families hypertension is common. While hereditary and genetic factors may be responsible, there is no doubt that the lifestyle of these families may be equally instrumental in keeping the blood pressure of its members at a high level. In the present stage of medical knowledge, nothing can be done to change the heredity of the members, but much can be achieved by indentifying the adverse factors in the lifestyle of hypertensive families and correcting them where correction is called for. The following adverse factors may be looked for:

- high consumption of common salt,
- highly spiced food with large content of chillies,
- liberal consumption of achars (pickles) and chutneys,
- low consumption of green vegetables,
- low consumption of fresh fruits,
- low consumption of milk, yoghurt and buttermilk (lassi),
- high consumption of animal foods, eggs and animal fats,
- high consumption of tobacco and alcohol,
- lack of physical activity and exercise, and
- overuse of auto-vehicles.

If the lifestyle of a hypertensive family includes several of the above factors, it needs to be altered not only in the interest of the hypertensive adults but also for the sake of the future health of the children. The adverse effects of unhealthy habits and food start early. It has been shown that factors which affect adult blood pressure are already operating in children. Studies have shown the importance of dietary salt, in relation to blood pressure, even in the first year of life. See chapter 20 for details.

19

Hypertension in Children

Hypertension in children is much less common than in adults. Unlike in adults, when detected in children, it is usually secondary to some other disease, of the kidneys, hormone glands, aorta, etc. Many of these abnormalities are inborn and some are amenable to surgical treatment, which may not only cure the disease but also the hypertension.

Essential Hypertension

Hypertension without a demonstrable cause is not common in children. The upper limit of normal blood pressure in children is 100/70 at the age of 1 year, rising to about 124/80 at age 13 and 130/84 at age 18. Though frank essential hypertension during childhood years is uncommon, an interesting recent study of blood pressure of school children and later when they became adults showed that adult blood pressure correlates with childhood blood pressure. The hypertensive adults had their childhood BP readings higher than what is considered normal at that age. Further, the hypertensive adults tend to be heavier and show the greatest increase in their weight from childhood. Prevention of fat acquisition during childhood, especially during the adolescent years, is now considered useful in preventing not only obesity but also hypertension in later years.

What You Should Do for Your Child's Hypertension

If your child's blood pressure is found to be consistently above the upper limit of normal for his age, you should get him investigated for any underlying cause, and if found, get it treated surgically, if necessary and feasible.

If no such cause is found, it may be a good idea to take the following simple measures, in addition to any treatment prescribed for him:

- reduce body weight, if obese; see Chapter 13(iv);
- give lacto-vegetarian diet in preference to a non-vegetarian diet;
- reduce salt intake to less than 1/3rd of normal consumption;
- give more potassium in the form of vegetables (legumes) and fruits, especially citrus and bananas;
- remove any cause of stress in school or at home;
- encourage active games and exercise;
- discourage excessive TV viewing; it raises the blood pressure;
- reduce his intake of saturated fats (eggs, butter, ghee);
- avoid giving junk food, e.g., highly salted potato chips, hamburgers, hot dogs;
- avoid smoking and alcohol yourself if you wish your child to abstain.

Emergencies

A diastolic pressure, due to any cause, above 95 mm in a small child or 110 mm in an older child is a matter of great concern as it can cause serious problems, including encephalopathy, brain haemorrhage and failure of the left ventricle of the heart. It needs urgent control.

Healthy Habits

Healthy habits are taught to the children by example. If you are anxious about the future health of your children and feel that their lifestyle and diet need to be improved, then you have to change the lifestyle and diet of the whole family and not merely attempt to change the children's. If such a diet is only made for the child, he will perceive that his diet is restricted and the parents' is not. This will only lead to tension and revolt or deceit. Ensure good health for yourself and the future health of your children by adopting a healthy lifestyle (Chapter 21) for the whole family.

20

When You Need to Consult Your Doctor

After the initial diagnosis and start of therapy by your physician, your spouse or someone else in the household should be checking your blood pressure regularly, say twice a week. The method of checking the blood pressure has already been explained in Chapter 4. After your spouse has learnt and practised the technique, get his/her readings checked by your doctor to make certain that his/her observations are reliable. Note the readings in a note-book to show to your physician on your next visit and for his future reference.

You need to consult the doctor under the following circumstances:

(A) For regular checks at intervals specified by him, say, three monthly, to enable him to:
- observe that your blood pressure is under good control;
- ensure that no complication of the disease is occurring; and to take timely action, if found;
- to detect any complication, he may occasionally need some investigations to be done;
- to suitably amend the dose of drug/s, if necessary, for optimal effect;
- to look for any undesirable side-effect of antihypertensive drug therapy, and take corrective action;

(B) Report to your doctor without waiting for the scheduled visit; if

- your blood pressure has gone out of control, either too high (above 160/100) or too low (below 120/80);
- there are spurts of hypertension;
- you feel unsteady on standing up; (it may be due to excessive fall of BP on standing);
- there is any somnolence, interfering with your work or driving;
- you experience frightening dreams (as with some betablockers) depressing thoughts of uselessness or suicide (as with Serpasil); change of drug is urgent;
- you experience severe weakness or cramps, which could be due to depletion of potassium by diuretics (try orange juice);
- there is any disturbance of sexual function; some of the antihypertensive drugs can cause problems like loss of libido and sexual potency. The problem is temporary; your doctor will identify the offending drug and change it.

Never miss on your dose or suddenly stop or change the treatment. It can cause a sudden severe rebound rise of blood pressure, which can end up in a catastrophe.

Some drugs cause first-dose hypotension. Your doctor will usually start with a small dose (unless there is an urgent need to lower the pressure) and will gradually build up the dose. In case, after starting a new drug you experience sudden severe weakness and pain in the legs or vertigo or loss of consciousness, your doctor must be informed, who will take the remedial action necessary.

(C) To immediate consultation with your doctor is necessary if you experience any of the following symptoms:

- bleeding from the nose—the blood pressure may be very high;
- sudden rise of blood pressure above 200/120;
- pain in the front of the chest at rest or on exertion;

- pain in the chest which is radiating to the shoulder, arm, neck or back or in any of these sites;
- sudden severe weakness, restlessness or cold sweats;
- laboured or difficult breathing at rest or on such exertion which did not produce the symptom before;
- sudden severe headache;
- convulsions;
- uselessness of arm or leg, even though it recovers after a few hours;
- paralysis.

21

Lifestyle for the Hypertensive

The management of hypertension is directed to one single goal—prevention of complications of the disease. The fundamental point is that whatever control of blood pressure is possible by physiological means without the use of drugs, that must be achieved, i.e., by increasing physical activity, losing weight, cutting down common salt and alcohol, stopping smoking and increasing consumption of vegetables and fruits. In mild cases such a course of action may obviate the necessity of drugs, and in the more severe cases it may reduce their need to the minimum.

While it must be emphasised that proper control of hypertension, with or without drugs, is of paramount importance, it has also to be admitted that all drugs are chemical substances and none can be assumed to be free from undesirable side-effects. Since they have to be taken by the patient on a life-long basis, the minimum possible amount is best, though that minimum amount should not be less than the effective dose. It is in this light that you have to view the lifestyle changes that have been suggested in this book. But for those who cannot maintain these changes or whose high blood pressure persists, drugs are added to protect their health. Keeping in view the above observations, following lifestyle is suggested for the hypertensive patient:

1. Food

- Low-salt diet:
  - prepare food without adding salt; daily ration of salt, to be used in any manner, allowed as under:

    for wheat-eaters : 2/3 teaspoon or less

    for rice-eaters : 1 teaspoon or less
  - salt need not be entirely cut out—deficiency of salt can be harmful in summer; increase by ½ teaspoon.
  - no red chillies in food; they need more salt for taste;
  - for dishes without gravy, just sprinkle salt but do not mix; it will be salty enough with half the amount of salt;
  - do not eat the gravy.
- Eat vegetarian food generally:
  - plenty of fresh green and leafy vegatables;
  - fresh fruits of the season;
  - pulses, according to your liking;
  - sparse use of pickles and chutneys.
- Eat non-vegetarian food occasionally: (Fish can be taken freely).
  - chicken and fowl in moderation;
  - avoid red meat (lamb, pork, beef);
  - abstain from organ meat (brain, liver, kidney, etc.).
- Consume milk and yoghurt (dahi), with most of the fat skimmed off.
- Cooking medium; any vegetable oil (not solidified).
- Ghee and butter, restricted.
- Eggs: 5 or less per week.
- Additional precautions for diabetics and obese:
  - avoid sugar, sweets or sweet dishes;
  - other carbohydrates, as allowed by the doctor;
  - restricted consumption of fats;
  - avoid fried food.

2. Beverages, Alcoholic

- Best to be a teetotaller.

- A peg is good for the BP and heart; more is poison.
- Maximum daily amount of spirits (whisky, brandy) admissible:
  - for men: 60 ml.
  - for women: 40 ml.
  - 2 alcohol-free days a week.

3. Beverages, Non-alcoholic (tea, coffee, cola drinks, chocolate)

- In moderation.
- 3-4 cups of tea and a cola drink or a cup of coffee in a day.

4. Tobacco

- Best avoided.
- If not possible to avoid, smoke pipe in strict moderation without deep inhaling.
- Do not chew tobacco, pan or pan masala.

5. Body Weight

- Maintain ideal weight; see chart (Appendix III).
- Do not have ups and downs of weight by losing and regaining; it is worse than being overweight.
- Diet, restricted for the obese (Appendix I).
- Exercise.
- Aim to reduce about 1½ kg per month, if obese.

6. Exercise

- Maintain a physically active life.
- Take regular, moderate exercise.
- If not used to exercise, don't rush into it; start with a small amount and gradually build up.
- Avoid exercise and strenuous physical work when the BP is inordinately high, or if adverse symptoms (chest pain, breathlessness, weakness) appear.

7. Stress

- Avoid, both physical and mental stress:
  - Keep your cool, avoid losing temper; not a muted response to aggression but a philosophical attitude.
  - Maintain regular hours of work, meals, rest and recreation without periods of sudden or excessive strain.
  - Do not work against time; avoid hurry; stop looking at watch too often; feel free, not time-bound.
  - Do not leave work in hand half done; this causes tension.
  - Face your problems squarely and strive to find solutions; unsolved problems build up tension.
  - Maintain a steady and moderate pace of life physically, mentally and emotionally without hurry and tension.
  - Do not force yourself to go on exerting in the face of any adverse symptoms, or when excessively tired or fagged out.
  - Avoid confrontations.
  - Use music, travel or hobbies as useful antidotes.
  - Have regular working holiday and 2 weeks vacation twice a year.
  - Keep an attitude of peaceful contentment.

8. Sexual Activity

- Keep up normal activity at a moderate pace.
- Clandestine activity can cause serious problems.
- If abnormal symptoms are precipitated, consult your physician.

9. Religion and Faith

- Faith is helpful in lowering blood pressure.
- Religious books and discourses are helpful, but only for those who have faith.

10. Meditation

- Meditation may help lower BP; learn the technique at a good meditation centre.

11. For Your Children

- Breast feed in preference to giving cow's milk or formula milk.
- Prevent acquisition of fat in the first two years of life and during adolescence by introducing prudent dietary habits from the beginning.
- Ensure low salt intake.

12. Pregnancy

- Do not smoke.
- Maintain good nutrition.
- Get anaemia treated, if present.
- Avoid all unnecessary drugs and medicines.
- Regular check of BP and urine albumin.

22

Prevention of Hypertension

Is it possible to prevent hypertension? Till very recently, we could not even think in those terms, much less ask such a question. Thanks to recent research, the possibility now appears to be in sight.

Having learnt about the various adverse factors which cause elevation of blood pressure and the associated metabolic abnormalities (Chapter 8), and more significantly, the importance of breast milk, and the fact that factors which operate in adult hypertension start operating as early as in the first year of life, I believe we are now in a position to form a strategy to prevent to a considerable extent not only hypertension but also obesity and diabetes in the later life of our children.

While it is quite possible that more factors of importance may come to light by future research, in the present stage of knowledge the following guidelines are suggested:

(1) Ensure a healthy intrauterine environment for the unborn child. The expectant mother should:
- ensure good nutrition during pregnancy and lactation;
- get anaemia treated, if present;
- abstain from smoking;
- avoid unnecessary drugs and medicines.

(2) Breast-feed the baby in preference to cow's milk or formula milk.
(3) Prevent obesity in early childhood by ensuring a proper diet.
(4) Take special care in diet in the first two years of life and again in adolescence as this is necessary to prevent acquisition of fat.
(5) Give a low salt diet from the beginning.
(6) Encourage regular exercise.
(7) Discourage excessive TV viewing by children.
(8) Teach the child healthy habits from the beginning by adopting a healthy lifestyle for the whole family (Chapter 20).

23

Some Questions and Their Answers

In this chapter I will answer a few questions which are commonly asked by patients. For details see relevant chapters of the book.

Q.1. What is normal BP?

A. 130/80 is considered normal BP. 140/90 is the upper limit of normal BP.

Q.2. What is high BP?

A. Above 140/90.

Q.3. What is optimum BP?

A. 120/80 for adults.

Q.4. What is low BP?

A. A habitually low BP, e.g., 100/70, in young people and not caused by any disease is a blessing; while a sudden fall due to a disease, e.g., a heart attack, even to a higher figure may cause alarm.

Q.5. Is there any effect of seasons on BP?

A. BP is usually higher in winter than in summer.
Loss of salt through perspiration in summer lowers BP, while constriction of peripheral blood vessels due to cold in winter elevates it.

Q.6. What are the symptoms of high BP?

A. Usually none.

Q.7. What about headache?

A. Headache is usually due to other factors like nervous

tension, which may raise the BP as well as cause the headache. However, a sudden rise of BP to very high levels, say, 200/120, may cause restlessness and headache directly.

Q. 8 Can high BP be familial?

A. Yes, hypertensive families exits.

Q. 9. What is the cause for familial high BP?

A. (i) Genetic factors;

(ii) the family's lifestyle and eating habits may be defective, e.g., consumption of highly salted food, alcohol, non-vegetarian food to the exclusion of vegetables and fruits; and

(iii) family tension.

Q. 10. It there any personality type which is prone to high BP?

A. Yes, the so-called type A personality—overambitious, pushing, working against time and obstacles.

Q.11. What is the effect of marital discord on BP?

A. Marital discord produces stress and tension which tends to raise BP.

Q.12. What happens if a hypertensive woman becomes pregnant?

A. The blood pressure treatment is suitably modified to drugs which are safe for the unborn child. With good blood pressure control, usually the pregnancy can go to term without problems unless toxaemia of pregnancy occurs in addition.

Q. 13. What happens if a previously normotensive woman has high blood pressure during pregnancy?

A. This may be due to toxaemia of pregnancy and is usually a serious matter both for the mother and the unborn child. The growth of the foetus may be retarded and stillbirth may occur. If the BP remains uncontrolled serious complications, including brain haemorrhage, may occur in the pregnent woman.

Q. 14. How is such a pregnancy treated?

A. Efforts are made to control the BP so as to take the pregnancy far enough for the foetus to be viable, i.e., it can live outside the mother. But if this is not possible, the foetus may have to be sacrificed to save the mother. As soon as the pregnancy is over or terminated, the blood pressure comes back to normal.

Q. 15. Is high BP contagious?

A. No.

Q. 16. What are the adverse effects of high BP?

A. Complications like angina, heart attacks, strokes, eye and kidney damage.

Q. 17. How many months' treatment cures high BP?

A. Unless hypertension is caused by some other disease, which is usually not the case, there is no cure but control.

Q. 18. Control, how long?

A. Lifelong control is essential to prevent serious complications. Therefore, treatment is lifelong.

Q.19. How does alcohol affect blood pressure?

A. Small quantities lower the BP. Regular consumption of large amounts is associated with increased incidence and worsening of hypertension.

Q. 20. How does smoking affect BP?

A. Though smoking raises the blood pressure only temporarily, it is a serious risk factor for the heart and so is hypertension. It is linked to so many other serious diseases like cancer of the lung. Hypertensives should, therefore, stop.smoking.

Q. 21. Are there any drugs which cause high BP?

A. Yes, e.g., corticosteroids, oral contraceptives, etc.

Q. 22. Can high BP cause psychological/personality changes?

A. By itself, high blood pressure does not cause such changes. However, if small blood clots occur in the arteries, of the brain as a result of prolonged hypertension, such changes can be produced.

Q. 23. Should a patient of hypertension restrict his activities?

A. If the blood pressure is well controlled, moderate physical activity is beneficial. It needs to be restricted only when the BP is inordinately high or if a complication like a heart attack occurs.

Q. 24. Are there any restrictions on sexual intercourse?

A. In uncomplicated hypertension, no restrictions need to be imposed if the BP is well controlled. In effect, sexual intercourse may be helpful in releasing tension. However, if complications like heart problems are present, such cases have to be individually assessed.

Q. 25. What are the precautions to be taken while taking antihypertensive drugs?

A. (i) Never stop medication abruptly;
(ii) never miss a dose,
(iii) when treatment is changed, watch out for first-dose excessive fall of BP with some drugs;
(iv) if excessive weakness, depression, frightening dreams or sexual weakness appear, report to your doctor for a change of drug or dosage.

Q. 26. Why are lifestyle changes necessary?

A. (i) They lower the BP;
(ii) they obviate the necessity of antihypertensive drugs or reduce their need and therefore, the dose;
(iii) they take care of any co-existing metabolic disturbances like high blood cholesterol;
(iv) they reduce obesity;
(v) they reduce incidence of complications of hypertension.

Q. 27. What are the necessary lifestyle changes?

A. Mainly they are:
(i) Low salt intake,
(ii) consumption of plenty of vegetables and fruits,

(iii) low intake of animal fats and high cholesterol foods,
(iv) avoidance/reduction of alcohol intake,
(v) avoidance of smoking,
(vi) weight reduction in case of obesity,
(vii) regular exercise,
(viii) avoidance of tension,
(ix) meditation, recreation, holiday.

Q. 28. How much salt should a hypertensive consume?

A. $^{2}/_{3}$ teaspoonful per day. This may be increased to one teaspoon in the case of a rice-eater.

Q. 29. Is it better to take a completely salt-free diet?

A. No, this can be dangerous in summer, especially if you are taking an oral diuretic, as there is much loss of salt through perspiration in summer.

Q. 30. Is a non-vegetarian diet harmful for the hypertensive?

A. No, except high cholesterol foods like organ meat and eggs. It is the exclusion of vegetables and fruits which is harmful.

Q. 31. Why is a vegetarian diet good for the hypertensives?

A. A vegetarian diet contains fibre, potassium, calcium and magnesium. All these elements lower the blood pressure. Also, it is free from saturated fats like cholesterol; therefore, it is more healthy for the heart.

Q. 32. How does one prevent hypertension?

A. (i) Ensure the health of the pregnant woman; she should be well nourished;
(ii) breast-feed the baby;
(iii) prevent obesity in early childhood and adolescence by ensuring healthy diet;
(iv) give a low salt diet to the child from the beginning;
(v) consume vegetarian food and fruits;
(vi) abstain from alcohol and smoking;
(vii) exercise regularly.

Q. 33. My father is aged 75 and hypertensive. At what level should his blood pressure be kept?

A. At around 150/92. The diastolic pressure should not fall much below 90 mm.

Q. 34. Is it safe for a hypertensive person to travel by air?

A. With modern pressurised aircrafts, air travel makes no difference to blood pressure. However, the distressing problems at the airport of customs clearance, immigration formalities and security checks, as well as any associated health problems like ischaemic heart disease should be taken into consideration while making plans for air travel, especially international. Of course, keep your blood pressure under good control while on the move.

Q. 35. What about vacation in the hills?

A. Going to an altitude of five or six thousand feet, where most of our hill stations are located, does not adversely affect the blood pressure, but keeps it well under control. You should stay where there are level walks nearby and not steep heights to climb. Any associated health problems, especially of the heart, should of course, be taken into consideration while planning a holiday in the hills.

24

Epilogue

In developed urbanised societies, life is more sedentary, obesity is common, intake of salt and alcohol is high and response to stress is often muted by social pressures. It is in populations with these characteristics that hypertension is common.

What is happening in developing countries like ours?

Industrialisation is occurring at a breakneck speed. People are on the move from rural to urban settings. Reports indicate not only a rising incidence of hypertension but also levels even higher than those reported in the developed countries. The phenomenon is associated with altered living patterns with a higher consumption of salt, smoking and drinking, greater stress and competition and major dietary changes resulting in both obesity and hypertension. In our country, vegetarians are turning to non-vegetarian foods, which are usually highly spiced and salted with a high content of fat. Vegetables and fruits, with their fibre and minerals, take a back seat. A sedentary life with over-use of cars and scooters and little physical activity and exercise complete the pattern of living which is now considered responsible for causing hypertension and its complications in those city-dwellers who have been so programmed either genetically or through adverse early environmental influences.

On the other hand, the vegetarian food without much salt and spice, with little fat and much fibre, which the villager was eating in his village, where there was no stress and little competition but lot of physical activity, kept his blood pressure normal.

The present-day trends of urbanisation and altered lifestyles are powerful. It is, therefore, necessary that the message of the adverse effects implicit in the altered living pattern, and in the abandoning of simple life and vegetarian food, reaches the urbanised masses widely to help them suitably improve their lifestyle. Parents should get anxious about lifestyle and future health of their children, with unambiguous commitment to inculcating healthy dietary habits and lifestyle for themselves and for their children. This will safeguard their own health as well as teach the children the value of healthy habits by setting an example to them, for children learn best by example.

It would be naive to suggest that the last word on hypertension has been said. Research on a global scale continues for more and more facts, and better and better drugs. Therefore, keep your mind open and receptive to new ideas.

I hope you have enjoyed reading this book, and more important, that you will find it useful. I must emphasize again that the treatment of hypertension is lifelong—without drugs if possible, with drugs if necessary.

I will look forward to your valuable suggestions and constructive criticism. You may write to me at this address: 7, Tribune Colony, Ambala Cantonment-133001 (Haryana), India.

25

Appendices

APPENDIX I

HINTS ON FOOD

1. Food for the Obese

(a) Consume freely:

- Beans, cabbage, cauliflower, carrots, cucumber, lettuce, mushrooms, onions, pumpkin, radish, spinach, turnip, brinjal, ladies' finger and gourds (tinda, gheea).
- Fruits (without added sugar): lemon, oranges, malta, melon, keenu, strawberries, raspberries, grapefruit, sweet lime.
- Tea or coffee (without sugar), soda water, lemon juice, tomato juice, diabetic fruit squash, clear unthickened soup, soup made of chicken or beef cubes.
- Artificial sweetening agents (such as saccharine), salt and pepper, vinegar, mustard, herbs, flavourings and colourings.

(b) Avoid consuming:

- Sugar, jaggery, gur, glucose.
- Sweets, toffees, chocolates, biscuits (chocolate and cream) and similar items of confectionery.
- Sweetmeats : Jalebi, gulab jaman, rasgulla, ras malai, burfi, peda, balushahi, etc.

- Sweet dishes: halwa, custard, firni, puddings
- Jams, marmalades, honey
- Tinned fruits, murabbas
- Dried fruits: dates, figs, apricot, sultanas (kishmish)
- Fruits (very sweet): mangoes, grapes (restricted use)
- Cakes, buns and pastries
- Cereals: rice, spaghetti, macaroni
- Breakfast cereals, porridge
- Beverages such as cocoa, Boost, Bournvita, Ovaltine
- Ice creams, fresh cream, fruit cream
- Condensed milk
- Nuts
- Salad cream, salad dressing, mayonnaise
- Thickened sauces
- Sweet pickles and chutneys
- Thickened soups and rich gravies
- Alcoholic drinks: beer, wines, sherry, spirits
- Sweetened fruit juices, fruit squash
- Cola drinks and other sweet fizzy drinks
- Sausages
- Butter, cream (malai), egg yolk, ghee, vegetable oil (except the minimum necessary for cooking)
- All fried food: parathas, samosas, pakoras, etc

Cook the food any way you like—by boiling, grilling, steaming, or baking, but do not fry or deep-fry in ghee or oil.

(c) All other foodstuffs not mentioned in lists (a) and (b) above, may be taken in moderation

2. Low Cholesterol Food

The cooking medium should be high in polyunsaturated fat content and low in saturated fats and cholesterol.

(a) Use:

- Polyunsaturated oil, e.g., sunflower oil, safflower oil, soyabean oil, corn oil or mustard oil, instead of ghee or animal fats as cooking medium.

- Polyunsaturated margarine instead of butter.

(b) Avoid:

- Butter
- Hydrogenated margarine and oils
- All animal fats: ghee, lard, suet
- Cakes, biscuits and pastries made with the above ingredients
- Sweetmeats made from animal fats
- Fatty meats and organ meats (brain, liver, kidney)
- Whole milk and cream
- Chocolates, ice-cream and fruit cream
- Cheese
- Coconut and coconut oil
- Eggs (yolk)
- Shellfish
- All fried foods.

3.Food for the Diabetic

(a) Avoid altogether:

- Sugar, glucose, jaggery (gur)
- Jams, marmalade, murabbas
- Syrups, sherbet and honey
- Tinned fruits
- Sweets like toffees and chocolates and halwai sweets
- Sweet biscuits, chocolate biscuits, cream biscuits
- Cola, lemonade and other sweet fizzy drinks, glucose drinks
- Sweetened milk preparations and condensed milk
- Cakes, pastries, pies, puddings and thick sauces
- Alcoholic drinks: beer, wines, spirit.

(b) Consume in moderation:

- Chapattis
- Bread, white or brown
- Biscuits (not sweet)
- Breakfast cereals and porridge (without sugar)

- All fresh and dried fruits
- Macaroni, spaghetti, custard, cornflour (without sugar)
- Thick soups
- Diabetic foods
- Milk and its products
- Pulses (dals)
- Egg (restricted consumption)
- Red meat (restricted consumption)
- Potatoes

(c) Consume freely:

- All white meat and fish
- Clear soups
- Meat extracts
- Tomato juice, lemon juice, orange juice
- Tea or coffee (without sugar)
- Fresh vegetables: cauliflower, spinach, turnip, brinjals, ladies's finger, gourds (tinda, gheea), French beans, onions, mushrooms, lettuce, cucumber, spring onions, radish, bitter gourd (karela), pea and beans
- Spices and herbs, salt, pepper and mustard
- Artificial sweetening agents such as saccharine, sugar-free.

For obese or overweight diabetics, all fats (animal or vegetable) should be restricted and fried foods in all forms should be banned.

Appendix II

SOURCES OF MINERALS IN FOOD

Since the presence of adequate quantities of potassium, magnesium and calcium in the diet is necessary to keep the blood pressure from rising, the sources from which these minerals are available are given below:

Potassium

- cereals
- fresh vegetables
- dried peas and beans
- fresh fruits, especially citrus, banana, water melon
- fruit juices (orange, malta, sweet lime)
- nuts
- molasses
- cocoa
- fresh fish and poultry
- beef and ham (restricted use for hypertensives)

Calcium

- milk and cheese
- cream and eggs (restricted use)

- cauliflower, beans, cabbage, carrots, lettuce, spinach, turnips, beetroot
- fruits such as dates, figs, pineapple, oranges
- bran, almonds, chocolate, oysters, shellfish

Magnesium

Widely distributed in foods specially :

- whole grain
- fruits
- vegetables.

Appendix III

DESIRABLE BODY WEIGHTS
(Minimum clothing : without shoes)

Height		Weight	
		Men	Women
in ft	in cm	in kg	in kg
4-10	148	—	48-51
4-11	150	—	49-52
5-00	153	—	51-54
5-01	156	—	52-55
5-02	158	56-60	53-57
5-03	161	58-62	54-58
5-04	163	59-64	56-60
5-05	166	61-65	58-61
5-06	168	62-67	59-64
5-07	171	64-69	61-65
5-08	173	66-71	62-67
5-09	176	68-73	64-69
5-10	178	69-74	66-70
5-11	181	71-76	67-72
6-00	184	73-79	69-74
6-01	186	75-81	—
6-02	189	78-84	—
6-03	191	80-86	—

Simplified Formula
for maximum desirable body weight

Men	5 ft	55 kg
Women	5 ft	52 kg

Add 2 kg per extra inch of height.

Glossary

Acute disease: a disease with severe symptoms, of rapid onset and short duration

Anaemia: a condition of blood with reduction of red blood cells or haemoglobin or both

Angina: full name angina pectoris; a heart pain of a few minutes' duration, usually located in the front of the chest

Angiography: X-ray of arteries after injection of a substance which is opaque to X-rays

Angioplasty: Plastic surgery on an artery, usually the coronary artery

Aorta: the largest artery of the body into which the heart pumps the blood and which distributes it to the whole body through its branches

Artery: a tube-like structure that carries blood from the heart to the tissues

Asthma: difficulty of breathing caused by spasm of the air tubes of the lungs due to allergy

Asthma, cardiac: an entirely different condition of difficulty of breathing due to dysfunction of the left ventricle of the heart

Atheroma: a plaque of fatty deposit on the wall of an artery

Atrophy: wasting or decrease in the size of a tissue

Blood vessel: artery or vein

C.A.D.: coronary artery disease (see under ischaemic heart disease)

Capillary: the thinnest blood vessel. Capillaries form network in tissues, from which the exchange of oxygen, carbon dioxide, water, salts, etc., between the blood and the tissues takes place

Carbohydrates: nutrients which are converted by the body to sugar (glucose) to produce energy (abundant in vegetarian food)

Cardiac, cardiological: pertaining to the heart

Cardiac arrest: sudden stoppage of heart action

Cardiac asthma: see asthma, cardiac

Catheter: a tube for insertion into a narrow opening

Cholesterol: a fatty substance present in animal fats, body tissues, and blood. HDL-cholesterol is a form beneficial for the heart and arteries, while LDL-cholesterol is the harmful form

Chronic disease: a disease of long duration, of gradual onset and slow progression, not acute

Coma : unrousable unconscious state

Contrast medium: a substance opaque to X-rays, so that an organ not visible in plain X-rays becomes visible

Coronary artery: the artery supplying blood to the heart

Coronary bypass operation: a shunt established surgically which permits blood to travel from the aorta to a coronary artery bypassing the obstruction in the latter

Debility: weakness

Diastolic blood pressure: the lowest reading of blood pressure on a blood pressure instrument, recorded when the ventricles are not contracting to produce the pulse beat

Diuretic: a drug which increases the volume of urine.

Encephalopathy, hypertensive: acute dysfunction of the brain due to very high blood pressure; it may cause temporary paralysis

Endocrine: a gland that manufactures hormones

Extrasystole: premature heartbeat

Foetus: the unborn child from the third month of pregnancy onwards

Gangrene: death and decay of a part of the body due to cessation of its blood supply

Genetic: pertaining to genes which carry inheritance

Gestation: pregnancy

Haemorrhage: bleeding, internal or external

Hemiplegia: paralysis of one side of the body

I.C.C.U.: intensive coronary care unit of a hospital

Hypertrophy: increase in the size of an organ

IHD: see ischaemic heart disease

Infarct: an area of dead tissue following cessation of its blood supply

Insulin: a hormone secreted by the pancreas; it metabolises sugar

Intrauterine life: life within the womb

Ischaemia: inadequate flow of blood to a part caused by obstruction to its blood supply

Ischaemic Heart Disease; **IHD, CAD**: narrowing and obstruction of the coronary artery due to fatty deposits, sufficient to prevent adequate blood supply to the heart, causing angina or heart attack

Left ventricular failure; left heart failure: failure of the function of the left ventricle, causing severe difficulty in breathing (cardiac asthma)

Lesion: an area of diseased tissue

Lipid: fat

Lumen: bore of an artery or vein

Metabolise: breakdown of food material by the body for energy production

Metabolism: the sum total of all chemical changes that take place within the body for maintenance of life, like energy production and body-building activity

Myocardial infarction: an acute heart attack; death of a part of the heart muscle following cessation of its blood supply

Necrosis: area of dead tissue surrounded by a healthy area

Nicotine: one the most toxic alkaloids found in tobacco

Parkinson's disease: a chronic nervous disease with fine tremors, rigidity and weakness of muscles and a mask-like face

Physiological: concerning the functions of the body

Pre-eclampsia: a condition which affects women in the advanced stage of pregnancy and is marked by high blood pressure, swelling of ankles and presence of protein in urine

Proteins: body-building substances in food; they are essential constituents of the body; presence of protein (albumin) in urine is a sign of kidney damage

Renal: pertaining to kidneys

Side-effects: unwanted, usually harmful, effects produced by a drug

Somnolence: drowsiness

Stress Test: method of evaluating the fitness of the heart by steadily increasing the level of exercise with simultaneous ECG to see changes produced by exercise

Stroke: sudden loss of consciousness followed by paralysis, caused by bleeding into the brain or clotting of blood in an artery of the brain

Systolic blood pressure: the highest reading of blood pressure recorded when the ventricles of the heart are contracting to produce the pulse beat

Thrombosis: formation of blood clot within an artery or vein

Tissue: a collection of similar cells which act together in the performance of a particular function, e.g., muscle, nerve

Vein: a tube-like structure that carries blood from the tissues back to the heart

Ventricles: two pumping chambers of the heart, the left and the right; the left one pumps blood into the aorta for distribution to the body; the right pumps blood into the lungs for oxygenation.

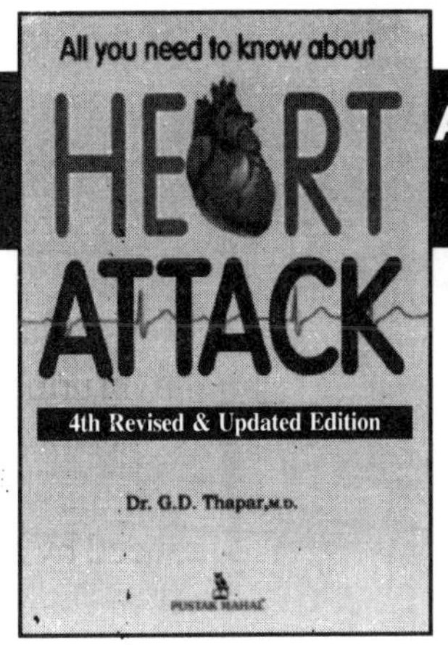

All you need to know about Heart Attack

—Dr. G.D. Thapar, M.D.

The following are some of the rare reviews received by the book.

This simply and concisely written book, aimed at the general public, contains useful information pertaining to heart attacks... The author must be praised for his simple, no-nonsense style of handling instructions pertaining to first-aid in cardiac arrest. Supported by good illustrations, the step-by-step instructions on mouth-to-mouth breathing and external cardiac massage make excellent reading.

—The Hindu

This book lives up to its title and describes a vast topic a comprehensive manner so that even a layman can understand and adopt certain preventive measures.

—The Tribune

Timely and useful... this book is an excellent source of information to which cardiologists may refer patients in health care and prevention of heart disease. Intelligent, informative and readable.

—Indian Review of Books

Demy size • Pages: 144
Price: Rs. 120/- • Postage: Rs. 15/-